Conquer Diabetes and Prediabetes

The Low-Carb Mediterranean Diet

Please visit us on the Internet at the Diabetic Mediterranean Diet blog:

http://DiabeticMediterraneanDiet.com

You'll find updated information and be able to interact with others interested in low-carb eating and diabetes.

Also by Steve Parker, M.D.:

The Advanced Mediterranean Diet: Lose Weight, Feel Better, Live Longer

http://AdvancedMediterraneanDiet.com

Advanced Mediterranean Diet Blog:
http://AdvancedMediterraneanDiet.com/blog/

Conquer Diabetes and Prediabetes

The Low-Carb Mediterranean Diet

Steve Parker, M.D.

扪文朽丘丹⻏七朽

First edition published 2011
ISBN 978-0-9791284-4-8
LCCN 2010932083

Published by pxHealth
PO Box 27276
Scottsdale, Arizona 85255 USA
Phone: (480) 695-3192
Web: http://pxHealth.com

Publisher's Cataloging-in-Publication data

Parker, Steven Paul.
    Conquer diabetes and prediabetes : the low-carb medi-
terranean diet / Steve Parker, M.D.
        p. cm.
    ISBN 978-0-9791284-4-8
    Includes bibliographical references and index.
    1. Diabetes --Diet therapy. 2. Weight loss. 3. Prediabetic
state –Prevention. 4. Obesity –Prevention 5. Insulin resistance --Diet therapy. 6. Low-carbohydrate diet. 7. Dietary
Carbohydrates --administration & dosage --Popular
Works. I. Title.

RC662 .P37 2011
616.4/620654 –dc22   2010932083

CONTENTS

Disclaimer
Dedication

Introduction   9

1   The Fundamentals   13

2   Normal Blood Sugars and Treatment Goals   21

3   Drugs for Diabetes   29

4   Hypoglycemia   55

5   Ketogenic Mediterranean Diet   63

6   Low-Carb Mediterranean Diet   81

7   A Week of Meals + Special Recipes   93

8   Daily Life With Very Low-Carb Eating   119

9   Prepare For Weight Loss   139

10   Exercise   157

11   Long-Term Maintenance   185

Additional Resources   191
Annotated Bibliography   195
Index   212

Disclaimer

The ideas and suggestions in this book are provided as general educational information only and should not be construed as medical advice or care. All matters regarding your health require supervision by a personal physician of other appropriate health professional familiar with your current health status. Always consult your personal physician before making any dietary, medication, or exercise changes. The publisher and author disclaim any liability or warranties of any kind arising directly or indirectly from the use of this book. If any problems develop, always consult your personal physician. Only your physician can provide you medical advice.

To my mother, Jean Murray Parker,
and to the memory of my father, Allan Edward
Parker (1927–2009)

Introduction

I'm sorry for what the medical establishment has done to people with diabetes.

We've done an atrocious job for type 2 diabetics and prediabetics.

We've recommended they eat precisely what their bodies can't handle: carbohydrates. We've urged them to take poison: carbohydrates. We've cooperated with the drug companies to encourage diabetics to eat foods that increase drug company profits: carbohydrates.

Much of the medical establishment's damage to diabetics has been done innocently, unknowingly. Rank and file physicians, dietitians, and nutritionists put blind faith in their instructors, scientific journal editors, and time-honored and tenured "thought leaders." Our unquestioning faith has hurt people with diabetes and prediabetes.

"But, Dr. Parker, you're too hard on doctors. Dietitians are the ones who tell diabetics what they should eat."

True, dietitians do an awful lot of dietary instruction. But physicians have much more training in chemistry, biochemistry, physiology, and disease processes. Doctors should have figured out long ago that standard diabetic diet advice was toxic. A few pioneering physicians indeed figured it out long before me. In chronological order, a few of the leaders are John Rollo (1797), Richard K. Bernstein, Richard C. Atkins, Mary C. Vernon, Michael R. Eades, Mary Dan Eades, and Eric Westman. Compared to the mainstream medical establishment, these doctors have had—unfortunately—insufficient influence among their colleagues.

Other physicians pioneered carbohydrate-restricted weight loss programs not necessarily focused on diabetes. Prominent names are Jean-François Dancel (French physician and surgeon, 1844), William Harvey (London, 1850s), Thomas Tanner (England, 1869), Frank Evans (Pittsburg, 1940s), Blake Donaldson (New York cardiologist, 1919), and Alfred Pennington (Delaware, 1940s)

For over two decades, I've been part of the problem, the mainstream medical establishment. But evidence accumulated over the last 10 years forces me to renounce my old ways. The scientific evidence, at first a trickle but now a tsunami, points to carbohydrate restriction as the best dietary approach to diabetes and prediabetes. *Major* carbohydrate restriction.

But set aside diabetes for a moment.

I've long been an advocate of the Mediterranean diet for the general population. It's well established that Mediterranean-style eating prolongs life and reduces the rates of numerous illnesses: heart attacks, strokes, cancer, dementia, and type 2 diabetes, for example.

It's also well established that having diabetes tends to shorten lifespan and promote heart attacks, strokes, and dementia. Several cancers are linked to diabetes: liver, pancreas, uterus, colon, breast, and bladder. The Mediterranean diet, remember, counteracts these scary trends. Why not combine carbohydrate restriction and the Mediterranean diet? You're about to see the world's first publically available eating plan that does just that: the Low-Carb Mediterranean Diet.

The most earth-shaking development in the field of nutrition over the last half century is the discovery that total fat and saturated fat in the diet are not particularly dangerous—if at all—for the vast majority of people. [For supporting documentation, see the Annotated Bibliography at the end of the book, or
http://advancedmediterraneandiet.com/blog/2009/07/06/are-saturated-fats-really-all-that-bad/.]

Carbohydrate-restricted diets have the potential to be relatively high in total and saturated fats. Until recently, total fat and saturated fat were thought to cause or contribute to atherosclerosis—hardening of the arteries—in turn leading to heart attacks, strokes, peripheral artery disease, and premature death.

Now that we know this theory is wrong, carbohydrate-restricted diets for weight management are in resurgence.

If you find out you're being poisoned, what's the first thing you do? Stop taking the poison, right? In this case, the poison is carbohydrates.

I've created a carbohydrate-restricted eating program that helps control diabetes. It helps resolve prediabetes or prevents progression to full-blown diabetes. It also reverses metabolic syndrome.

Yes, for too long the medical establishment has let down the diabetes community. This book is an effort to set things right.

1

The Fundamentals

Type 2 diabetes and prediabetes are epidemics because of excessive consumption of refined sugars and starches, and lack of physical activity.

SCOPE OF THE PROBLEM

Diabetes is the most important public health problem in the U.S. and most of the developed world. The U.S. Centers for Disease Control and Prevention predicts that one of every three Americans born in the year 2000 will develop diabetes.

The most common form of diabetes by far is type 2, which describes at least 85% of cases. It's less serious than type 1 diabetes. Type 1 diabetics have an immune system abnormality that destroys the pancreas's ability to make insulin. Type 1's will not last long without insulin injections. On the other hand, many type 2 diabetics live well without insulin shots.

The epidemic of diabetes in the U.S. and the developed world overwhelmingly involves type 2, not type 1. The focus of this book is type 2 diabetes and prediabetes.

"Prediabetes" is what you'd expect: a precursor that may become full-blown diabetes over time. Blood sugar levels are above average, but not yet into the diabetic range. One in four people with prediabetes develops type 2 diabetes over the course of three to five years. Researchers estimate that 30% of the adult U.S. population had prediabetes in 2006. That's one out of every three adults. Only 7% of them (less than one in 10) were aware they had it.

The rise of diabetes parallels the increase in overweight and obesity, which in turn mirrors the prominence of refined sugars and starches throughout our food supply. These trends are intimately related. Public health authorities 40 years ago convinced us to cut down our fat consumption in a mistaken effort to help our hearts. We replaced fats with body-fattening carbohydrates that test the limits of our pancreas to handle them. Diabetics and prediabetics fail that test.

Dr. Richard K. Bernstein, notable diabetologist, wrote that, "Americans are fat largely because of sugar, starches, and other high-carbohydrate foods."

In the U.S. as of 2008, 24 million adults have diabetes. That's 11% of all adults and 23% of those over 60. Another 57 million in the U.S. have prediabetes: one out of every three adults.

We're even starting to see type 2 diabetes in children, which was quite rare just thirty years ago. It's undoubtedly related to overweight and obesity. Childhood obesity in the U.S. tripled from the early 1980s to 2000, ending with a 17% obesity rate. Overweight and obesity together describe 32% of U.S. children.

Diabetes is important because it has the potential to damage many different organ systems, deteriorating quality of life. It can damage nerves (neuropathy), eyes (retinopathy), kidneys (nephropathy), and stomach function (gastroparesis), just to name a few.

Just as important, diabetes can cut life short. Compared to those who are free of diabetes, having diabetes at age 50 more than doubles the risk of developing cardiovascular disease—heart attacks, strokes, and high blood pressure. Compared to those without diabetes, having both cardiovascular disease and diabetes approximately doubles the risk of dying. Compared to those without diabetes, women and men with diabetes at age 50 die seven or eight years earlier, on average.

Diabetic complications and survival rates will improve over the coming decades as we learn how to better treat this ancient disease.

WHAT'S WRONG WITH DIABETICS?

The problem in type 2 diabetes and prediabetes is that the body cannot handle ingested carbohydrates in the normal fashion. In a way, dietary carbohydrates (carbs) have become toxic instead of nourishing. This is a critical point, so let's take time to understand it.

NORMAL DIGESTION AND CARBOHYDRATE HANDLING

The major components of food are proteins, fats, and carbohydrates. We digest food either to get energy, or to use individual components of food in growth, maintenance, or repair of our own body parts.

We need some sugar (also called glucose) in our bloodstream at all times to supply us with immediate energy. "Energy" refers not only to a sense of muscular strength and vitality, but also to fuel for our brain, heart, and other automatic systems. Our brains especially need a reliable supply of bloodstream glucose.

In a normal, healthy state, our blood contains very little sugar—about a teaspoon (5 ml) of glucose. [We have about one and a third gallons (5 liters) of blood circulating. A normal blood sugar of 100 mg/dl (5.56 mmol/l) equates to about a teaspoon of glucose in the bloodstream.]

Our bodies have elaborate natural mechanisms for keeping blood sugar normal. They work continuously, a combination of adding and removing sugar from the bloodstream to keep it in a healthy range (70 to 140 mg/dl, or 3.9 to 7.8 mmol/l). These homeostatic mechanisms are out of balance in people with diabetes and prediabetes.

By the way, glucose in the bloodstream is commonly referred to as "blood sugar," even though there are many other types of sugar other than glucose. In the U.S., blood sugar is measured in units of milligrams per deciliter (mg/dl), but other places measure in millimoles per liter (mmol/l).

When blood sugar levels start to rise in response to food, the pancreas gland—its beta cells, specifically—secrete insulin into the bloodstream to keep sugar levels from rising too high. The insulin drives the excess sugar out of the blood, into our tissues. Once inside the tissues' cells, the glucose will be used as an immediate energy source or stored for later use. Excessive sugar is stored either as body fat or as glycogen in liver and muscle.

When we digest fats, we see very little direct effect on blood sugar levels. That's because fat contains almost no carbohydrates. In fact, when fats are eaten with high-carb foods, it tends to slow the rise and peak in blood sugar you would see if you had eaten the carbs alone.

Ingested protein can and does raise blood sugar, usually to a mild degree. As proteins are digested, our bodies can make sugar (glucose) out of the breakdown products. The healthy pancreas releases some insulin to keep the blood sugar from going too high.

In contrast to fats and proteins, carbohydrates in food cause significant—often dramatic—rises in blood sugar. Our pancreas, in turn, secretes higher amounts of insulin to prevent excessive elevation of blood glucose. Carbohydrates are easily digested and converted into blood sugar. The exception is fiber, which is indigestible and passes through us unchanged.

During the course of a day, the pancreas of a healthy person produces an average of 40 to 60 units of insulin. Half of that insulin is secreted in response to meals, the other half is steady state or "basal" insulin. The exact amount of insulin depends quite heavily on the amount and timing of carbohydrates eaten. Dietary protein has much less influence. A pancreas in a healthy person eating a very-low-carb diet will release substantially less than 50 units of insulin a day.

To summarize thus far: dietary carbs are the major source of blood sugar for most people eating "normally." Carbs are, in turn, the main cause for insulin release by the pancreas, to keep blood sugar levels in a safe, healthy range.

Hang on, because we're almost done with the basic science!

CARBOHYDRATE HANDLING IN DIABETES & PREDIABETES

Type 2 diabetics and prediabetics absorb carbohydrates and break them down into glucose just fine. Problem is, they can't clear the glucose out of the bloodstream normally. So blood sugar levels are often in the elevated, poisonous range, leading to many of the complications of diabetes.

Remember that insulin's primary function is to drive blood glucose out of the bloodstream, into our tissues, for use as immediate energy or stored energy (as fat or glycogen).

In diabetes and prediabetes, this function of insulin is impaired.

The tissues have lost some of their sensitivity to insulin's action. This critical concept is called *insulin resistance*. Insulin still has some effect on the tissues, but not as much as it should. Different di-

18

abetics have different degrees of insulin resistance, and you can't tell by just looking.

Insulin resistance occurs in most cases of type 2 diabetes and prediabetes. So what causes the insulin resistance? In many cases it's related to overweight, physical inactivity, and genetics. A high-carbohydrate diet may contribute. A few cases are caused by drugs. Some cases are a mystery.

To overcome the body tissue's resistance to insulin's effect, the pancreas beta cells pump even more insulin into the bloodstream, a condition called hyperinsulinemia. Some scientists believe high insulin levels alone cause some of the damage associated with diabetes. Whereas a healthy person without diabetes needs about 50 units of insulin a day, an obese non-diabetic needs about twice that to keep blood sugars in check. Eventually, in those who develop diabetes or prediabetes, the pancreas can't keep up with the demand for more insulin to overcome insulin resistance. The pancreas beta cells get exhausted and start to "burn out." That's when blood sugars start to rise and diabetes and prediabetes are easily diagnosed. So, insulin resistance and high insulin production have been going on for years before diagnosis. By the time of diagnosis, 50% of beta cell function is lost.

Did you know that people who work at garbage dumps, sewage treatment plants, and cattle feedlots get used to the noxious fumes after a while? They aren't bothered by them as much as they were at first. Their noses are less sensitive to the fumes. You could call it fume resistance. In the same fashion, cells exposed to high insulin levels over time become resistant to insulin.

EXTRA CREDIT FOR INQUISITIVE MINDS

You've learned that insulin's main action is to lower blood sugar by transporting it into the cells of various tissues. But that's not all insulin does. It also 1) impairs breakdown of glycogen into glucose, 2) stimulates glycogen formation, 3) inhibits formation of new glucose molecules by the body, 4) promotes storage of triglycerides in fat cells (i.e., lipogenesis, fat accumulation), 5) promotes formation of fatty acids (triglyceride building blocks) by the liver, 6) inhibits breakdown of stored triglycerides, and 7) supports body protein production.

In his fascinating book, *Cheating Destiny: Living With Diabetes, America's Biggest Epidemic*, James Hirsch describes what happened to type 1 diabetics before insulin injections were available. Type 1 diabetics, remember, produce no insulin. Until Frederick Banting and Charles Best isolated and injected insulin in the 1920s, type 1 diabetes was a death sentence characterized not only by high blood sugars, but also extreme weight loss as muscle and fat tissue wasted away. The tissue wasting reflects insulin actions No.4, 5, 6, and 7 above.

Banting and Best worked at the University of Toronto in Canada. Their "discovery" of insulin is one of the greatest medical achievements of all time.

2

Normal Blood Sugars and Treatment Goals

Physicians focus so much on disease that we sometimes lose sight of what's healthy and normal. For instance, the American Diabetes Association defines "tight control" of diabetes to include sugar levels as high as 179 mg/dl (9.94 mmol/l) when measured two hours after a meal. In contrast, young adults without diabetes two hours after a meal are usually in the range of 90 to 110 mg/dl (5.00–6.11 mmol/l).

WHAT IS A NORMAL BLOOD SUGAR LEVEL?

The following numbers refer to average blood sugar (glucose) levels in venous plasma, as measured in a lab. Portable home glucose meters measure sugar in capillary whole blood, as opposed to venous plasma. Many meters in 2011—but not all—are calibrated to compare directly to venous plasma levels.

Average Blood Sugar Values Before and After a Meal:

Fasting blood sugar after a night of sleep and before breakfast: 85 mg/dl (4.72 mmol/l)

One hour after a meal: 110 mg/dl (6.11 mmol/l)

Two hours after a meal: 95 mg/dl (5.28 mmol/l)

Five hours after a meal: 85 mg/dl (4.72 mmol/l)

(The aforementioned numbers reflect a meal deriving 50–55% of its calories from carbohydrate—a typical carbohydrate percentage.)

***Ranges* of Blood Sugar for Young Healthy Non-Diabetic Adults:**

Fasting blood sugar: 70–90 mg/dl (3.89–5.00 mmol/l)

One hour after a typical meal: 90–125 mg/dl (5.00–6.94 mmol/l)

Two hours after a typical meal: 90–110 mg/dl (5.00–6.11 mmol/l)

Five hours after a typical meal: 70–90 mg/dl (3.89–5.00 mmol/l)

WHAT LEVEL OF BLOOD SUGAR DEFINES DIABETES?

According to the 2007 guidelines issued by the American Association of Clinical Endocrinologists:

Diabetes: fasting blood sugar 126 mg/dl (7 mmol/l) or greater

Diabetes: blood sugar 200 mg/dl (11.11 mmol/l) or greater two hours after ingesting 75 grams of glucose

Diabetes: random ("casual") blood sugar 200 mg/dl (11.11 mmol/l) or greater, plus symptoms of diabetes

If there's any doubt about the diagnosis, testing should be repeated on a subsequent day.

WHAT LEVEL OF BLOOD SUGAR DEFINES PREDIABETES?

According to the 2007 guidelines issued by the American Association of Clinical Endocrinologists:

Prediabetes: (or *impaired fasting glucose*): fasting blood sugar 100–125 mg/dl (5.56–6.94 mmol/l)

Prediabetes: (or *impaired glucose tolerance*): blood sugar 140–199 mg/dl (7.78–11.06 mmol/l) two hours after ingesting 75 grams of glucose

If there's any doubt about the diagnosis, testing should be repeated on a subsequent day.

Compared to impaired fasting glucose, impaired glucose tolerance may be a better predictor of cardiovascular disease and death. So some researchers and clinicians focus on preventing high blood sugar swings after meals.

The problem with prediabetes, which causes no symptoms early on, is that one of every four cases progresses to full-blown diabetes over the next three to five years.

The numbers above do not apply to pregnant women. Blood sugars tend to be a bit lower in pregnant women. Five out every hundred pregnant women in the U.S. develop *gestational diabetes* that goes away soon after delivery.

WHAT LEVEL OF HEMOGLOBIN A1C DEFINES DIABETES AND PREDIABETES?

Another way to consider normal and abnormal blood sugar levels is to look at a blood test called hemoglobin A1c, which is an indicator of average blood sugar readings over the prior three months. The average healthy non-diabetic adult hemoglobin A1c is 5% and translates into an average blood sugar of 100 mg/dl (5.56 mmol/l). This will vary a bit from lab to lab. Most healthy non-diabetics would be under 5.7%.

Hemoglobin A1c can be used to estimate average blood sugar levels over the preceding three months. First, remember that a hemoglobin A1c of 5% equals an average blood sugar of 100 mg/dl (5.56 mmol/l). For each one % higher than 5%, average glucose is approximately 40 mg/dl (2.22 mmol/l) higher than 100 mg/dl. For example, if hemoglobin A1c measures as 7%, it suggests that blood sugars have averaged 180 mg/dl (10 mmol/l) for the last three months.

In December, 2009, the American Diabetes Association established a hemoglobin A1c criterion for the diagnosis of diabetes: 6.5% or higher. Diagnosis of prediabetes involves hemoglobin A1c in the range of 5.7 to 6.4%. Alternatively, the aforementioned blood sugar criteria can also be used to make the diagnosis.

WHAT ARE BLOOD SUGAR AND HEMOGLOBIN A1C GOALS DURING TREATMENT FOR DIABETES?

The 2007 guidelines of the American Association of Clinical Endocrinologists "encourage patients to achieve glycemic levels as near normal as possible without inducing hypoglycemia." In other words, they recommend both type 2 and type 1 diabetics aim for sugars as close to normal as possible without causing *low* blood sugars. Specifically:

Fasting Blood Sugar: under 110 mg/dl (6.11 mmol/l)

Two Hours After a Meal: under 140 mg/dl (7.78 mmol/l)

Hemoglobin A1c: 6.5% or less

The American Diabetes Association in 2011 recommends normal or near-normal blood sugar levels, and defines "tight control" as:

Pre-Meal and Fasting Glucose Levels: 70–130 mg/dl (3.9–7.2 mmol/l)

Two Hours After Start of a Meal: under 180 mg/dl (10.00 mmol/l)

Hemoglobin A1c: under 7%

A hemoglobin A1c of 7% is equivalent to average blood sugar levels of 160 mg/dl (8.89 mmol/l). Hemogobin A1c of 6% equals, roughly, average blood sugar levels of 130 mg/dl (7.22 mmol/l). But remember, healthy non-diabetics spend most of their day under 100 mg/dl (5.56 mmol/l) and have hemoglobin A1c's around 5%.

Diabetes experts actively debate how tightly we should control blood sugar levels. For instance, Dr. Richard K. Bernstein—a type 1 diabetic himself—recommends keeping blood sugar levels under 90 mg/dl (5.00 mmol/l) almost all the time. If it exceeds 95 mg/dl (5.28 mmol/l) after a meal, then a change in medication or meal is in order, he says.

Here's the over-simplified "tight control" debate. On one hand, tight control helps prevent and may reverse some of the devastating consequences of diabetes, such as nerve damage, eye damage, and kidney disease. On the other hand, tight control in diabetics on insulin and certain other diabetic medications may raise the risk of life-threatening hypoglycemia and may shorten lifespan in other ways.

BLOOD SUGAR GOALS FOR MY PERSONAL DIABETIC AND PREDIABETIC PATIENTS

Ideally, in general, I like to see normal glucose levels before and after meals, with normal hemoglobin A1c.

Realistically, these are acceptable fall-back positions:

Fasting Blood Sugar: under 100 mg/dl (5.56 mmol/l)

One Hour After Meals: under 150 mg/dl (8.33 mmol/l)

Two Hours After Meals: under 130 mg/dl (7.22mmol/l)

Hemoglobin A1c: 6% or less

Admittedly, these goals are not acceptable or achievable by everyone with diabetes. Nor are they necessary for every diabetic. Goals should be customized and negotiable. My goals for a demented 88-year-old on dialysis (artificial kidney treatments) are not the same as for an otherwise healthy 45-year-old.

Treatment options for those not at goal include diet modification, weight loss, exercise, and medications.

Future studies may prove that such strict goals are not necessary to avoid the complications and premature death suffered by people with diabetes. Tight control may be less important for elderly diabetics over 65–70. But for now, if I were a young or middle-aged diabetic I'd shoot for the goals above.

EXTRA CREDIT: TECHNICAL NOTES

The gold standard for measuring glucose is a large chemistry analyzer machine in a lab, which measures values in plasma obtained from a *vein* with a needle. The glucose level in *capillary* whole blood, obtained via finger prick and analyzed on a portable/home glucose monitor, is a different value, often 5–10 mg/dl (0.28–0.56 mmol/l) higher than venous glucose. As of 2011, a majority of home glucose monitors—but not all—are calibrated so as to be directly comparable to venous plasma glucose readings. Read your monitor's paperwork to find out about your device.

Portable finger-stick glucose meters are not as accurate and as you might expect. If your actual glucose level is 100 mg/dl (5.56 mmol/l), the meter may report it as 80 or 120 mg/dl (4.43 or 6.67 mmol/l) or anywhere in between, for example. That's if all other conditions are perfect: your technique, storage of the test strips since they left the factory, proper function of the machine, etc. The meters tend to be less accurate at glucose values over 200 mg/dl (11.1 mmol/l). Some devices are definitely more accurate than others. Do your research on the available monitors before you acquire one.

Outside the U.S., glucose is usually reported in units of mmol/l (millimoles per liter). One mmol/l = 18 mg/dl. To convert mg/dl to mmol/l, divide by 18 or multiply by 0.055.

3

Drugs for Diabetes

We've never had so many pharmaceutical options for treating diabetes—11 different classes as of early 2011. Many classes have more than one drug. All classes available in the U.S. are discussed below.

We're reviewing drugs now in preparation for the next chapter, which is about low blood sugar, otherwise known as hypoglycemia. Diabetes medications are the major cause of hypoglycemia in people with diabetes. Blood sugars can drop dangerously low in people taking certain medications while cutting back on calorie consumption or reducing the amount of carbohydrates they eat. The more severe the carb restriction, the greater the risk of hypoglycemia.

WARNING!

THIS CHAPTER WILL PUT SUSCEPTIBLE INDIVIDUALS TO SLEEP. DO NOT OPERATE DANGEROUS MACHINERY OR DRIVE WHILE READING.

If you don't take any drugs to control diabetes or prediabetes, you're free to skip this chapter. Otherwise, find your drugs herein and pay careful attention to those. Reading about the other drugs is likely to bore you; skip them. Note especially if your drugs are the ones that can cause low blood sugar. If so, you and your doctor will have to reduce the medication dose—or even stop the drug—when you start the very-low-carb Ketogenic Mediterranean Diet. The next chapter has some tips on reducing drug dosages.

If you don't know your diabetic drug's name(s), go check the bottle now. Your pharmacist and personal physician are indispensible if any doubts remain about your drug's name, class, or potential to cause hypoglycemia.

I recommend you become the expert on the diabetic drugs you take. Don't depend solely on your physician. Do research at reliable sources and keep written notes. With a little effort, you could quickly surpass your doctor's knowledge of your specific drugs. What are the side effects? How common are they? How soon do they work? Any interactions with other drugs? What's the right dose, and how often can it be changed? Do you need blood tests to monitor for toxicity? How often? Who absolutely should not take this drug? Along with everything else your doctor has to keep up with, he prescribes about a hundred drugs on a regular basis. You only have to learn about two or three. It could save your life.

Be aware that drugs have both generic and brand names. For instance, metformin (a generic name) is sold under the brand name of Glucophage, among other brand names depending on the manufacturer. Complicating matters further is that generic and brand names vary from one country to the next. I practice medicine in the U.S., so U.S. names are the ones I'll use. I will always capitalize a brand name drug, but start generic names with lower case letters unless it's the first word of a sentence.

The U.S. Food and Drug Administration is charged with approving drugs as safe and effective, and monitoring ongoing safety once a drug is on the market. Doctors commonly prescribe drugs for purposes not approved by the FDA. That's called "off-label." However, for our purposes here, I've restricted my comments to FDA-approved uses.

I strive to be as accurate as possible in sharing drug information with you, but I cannot guarantee accuracy. Anything I write today could be outdated tomorrow. Talk to your personal physician, pharmacist, or other qualified professional for detailed, up-to-date drug information.

LIST OF DRUG CLASSES

DRUGS FOR TYPE 1 DIABETES

Insulins
Pramlintide: Symlin

DRUGS FOR TYPE 2 DIABETES

Metformin: Glucophage, others
Sulfonylureas: glipizide, glyburide, glimiperide, others

31

Thiazolidinediones: rosiglitazone (Avandia) pioglitazone (Actos)
Dipeptidyl-peptidase-4 Inhibitors: sitagliptin (Januvia), saxagliptin (Onglyza), vildagliptin
GLP-1 Analogues: exenatide (Byetta), liraglutide (Victoza)
Insulins
Alpha-glucosidase Inhibitors: acarbose (Precose), miglitol (Glyset)
Meglitinides: repaglinide (Prandin), nateglinide (Starlix)
Pramlintide: Symlin
Colesevelam: WelChol
Dopamine Receptor Agonist: bromocriptine (Cycloset)

INJECTABLE DRUGS FOR DIABETES

Insulins
Pramlintide: Symlin
GLP-1 Analogues: exenatide (Byetta), liraglutide (Victoza)

ORAL DRUGS (taken by mouth) FOR DIABETES

Metformin: Glucophage, others
Sulfonylureas: glipizide, glyburide, glimiperide, others
Thiazolidinediones: rosiglitazone (Avandia), pioglitazone (Actos)
Dipeptidyl-peptidase-4 Inhibitors: sitagliptin (Januvia), saxagliptin (Onglyza), vildagliptin
Alpha-glucosidase Inhibitors: acarbose (Precose), miglitol (Glyset)
Meglitinides: repaglinide (Prandin), nateglinide (Starlix)
Colesevelam: WelChol
Dopamine Receptor Agonist: bromocriptine

(Cycloset)

Now let's look at the specific drug classes.

ALPHA-GLUCOSIDASE INHIBITORS

Alpha-glucosidase inhibitors (AGIs) available in the U.S. are acarbose (Precose) and miglitol (Glyset).

How do they work?

Many of the carbohydrates we eat are just basic sugar molecules joined to each other by chemical bonds, creating disaccharides, oligosaccharides, and polysaccharides. This is as true for bread and potatoes as it is for table sugar. To digest and absorb them, we have to break them down into the basic sugar molecules (monosaccharides). AGIs inhibit this breakdown process inside our intestine, decreasing the expected rise in blood sugar after we eat carbohydrates composed of chains of basic sugar molecules. They delay glucose absorption. So AGIs mainly decrease after-meal glucose levels.

Uses

They work alone or in combination with other diabetic medications, especially if the diet contains over 50% of energy in the form of complex carbohydrates. They are FDA-approved only for use in type 2 diabetes, but they have also been used in type 1.

Dosing

The starting dose is the same for both: 25 mg by mouth three times daily with the first bite of each main meal.

Side Effects

Belly pain, intestinal gas, diarrhea. Slight risk of hypoglycemia when it's used alone; higher risk when used with insulin shots or insulin secretagogues. If hypoglycemia occurs, you have to eat glucose to counteract it, not your usual non-glucose items because you won't absorb them properly.

Don't Use If You Have . . .

. . . liver cirrhosis (don't use acarbose; miglitol is OK), kidney impairment, or intestinal problems.

BROMOCRIPTINE

Cycloset (bromocriptine mesylate) is the most recent drug approved for treatment of type 2 diabetes by the U.S. Food and Drug Administration. It's a completely new approach that increases dopamine activity in the brain.

Bromocriptine has been in use for many years to treat other conditions, so we may not see any of the unforeseen consequences that have led to so many drugs being pulled from the market a few years after FDA approval.

Class

Dopamine receptor agonist (the only drug in this class).

How Does It Work?

How it lowers glucose levels is not entirely clear, but it may reset or alter glucose metabolism in tissues outside the brain. Bromocriptine is an ergot derivative that increases dopamine activity in the brain. It improves after-meal glucoses without an increase in blood insulin levels. This is appealing since high insulin levels are implicated as a contributor to some chronic diseases.

Uses

It's for adults with type 2 diabetes and can be used alone or with certain other diabetes drugs. "Other drugs" used in clinical trials were mostly metformin and sulfonylureas, with less experience using it with thiazolidinediones. We know little about using it with insulin. Bromocriptine is not for type 1 diabetics or diabetic ketoacidosis. It lowers hemoglobin A1c by 0.6 to 0.9% (absolute decrease).

Dosing

Start with 0.8 mg every morning and increase by an additional tablet (0.8 mg) weekly up to 4.8 mg or the maximal tolerated dose (1.6 to 4.8 mg). Take all of it in the morning.

Side Effects

In clinical studies, the most common cause for discontinuation of the drug was nausea. It can cause drowsiness, fainting, blood pressure drops with standing (causing lightheadedness, fainting, weakness, or sweating), fatigue, vomiting, and headaches. Hypoglycemia is not much of a problem, if any, when bromocriptine is used as the sole diabetic medication. In other words, bromocriptine by itself may slightly increase the risk of hypoglycemia.

Don't Use It If You ...

. . . take neuroleptic drugs, are a nursing mother, have syncopal migraines (that make you faint), have hypersensitivity to ergot-related drugs, or have a severe psychotic disorder.

COLESEVELAM

Colesevelam is used primarily to reduce elevated levels of LDL cholesterol. It's sold in the U.S. as WelChol.

Class

Bile acid sequestrant.

How does it work?

Unclear.

Uses

Colesevelam is FDA-approved for treatment of type 2 diabetes in conjunction with insulin or diabetic pills.

Dosing

Three tablets twice daily with meals, or six tablets once daily with a meal.

Side Effects

Constipation in one of every 10 users.

Do Not Use If You Have . . .

. . . serum triglycerides over 500 mg/dl, or have gastroparesis, other gastrointestinal motility disorders, risk factors for bowel obstruction, or recent major gastrointestinal procedures.

DIPEPTIDYL-PEPTIDASE-4 INHIBITORS

The two dipeptidyl-peptidase-4 inhibitors available in the U.S. are sitagliptin (sold as Januvia) and saxagliptin (sold as Onglyza). Vildagliptin is available in other countries. Let's just call this class DPP-4 inhibitors.

How Do They Work?

DPP-4 inhibitors decrease both fasting and after-meal blood sugar levels primarily by increasing insulin release from pancreas beta cells. How they do it is complicated.

First off, you need to know that two gastrointestinal hormones levels—glucagon-like peptide-1 (GLP-1) and gastric inhibitory polypeptide—increase in response to a meal. These hormones increase insulin secretion by pancreas beta cells, suppress glucagon secretion from pancreas alpha cells after meals, help suppress glucose production by the liver, and improve glucose uptake by tissues outside the liver. GLP-1 also slows emptying by the stomach and reduces food intake. All this tends to lower glucose levels after meals.

Did I mention it was complicated?

If we could make these gut hormones hang around longer, their glucose-lowering action would be enhanced. How can we make them hang around and work longer? Simply suppress the enzyme that degrades them: dipeptidyl-peptidase-4. That's what DPP-4 inhibitors do.

The small intestine hormone GLP-1 is a major player in normal carbohydrate metabolism. GLP-1 levels, by the way, are decreased in type 2 diabetes.

For the DPP-4 inhibitors, we have no data on long-term safety, mortality, or diabetic complications.

Uses

Sitagliptin is FDA-approved as initial drug therapy for the treatment of type 2 diabetes, and as a second agent in those who do not respond to a single agent, such as metformin, a sulfonylurea, or a thiazolidinedione. It can also be used as a third agent when dual therapy with a sulfonylurea and metformin doesn't provide adequate blood sugar control.

Saxagliptin is FDA-approved as initial drug therapy for the treatment of type 2 diabetes or as an add-on drug for those who do not respond to a single drug, such as metformin, a sulfonylurea, or a thiazolidinedione.

Dosing

The DPP-4 inhibitors are given by mouth. The usual dose of sitagliptin is 100 mg once daily, with reduction to 50 mg in those with moderate to severe kidney impairment, and 25 mg for severe kidney impairment. The usual dose of saxagliptin is 2.5 or 5 mg once daily, with the 2.5 mg dose recommended for patients with moderate to severe kidney impairment.

Side Effects

Generally well-tolerated. No risk of hypoglycemia when used as the sole diabetes drug. They do not cause weight gain. Sitagliptin might cause pancreatitis.

Don't Use If You Have . . .

. . . moderate or severe kidney impairment (sitagliptin) or severe kidney impairment (saxagliptin). Use sitagliptin with caution and careful monitoring if you have a history of pancreatitis.

GLP-1 ANALOGUES

GLP-1 analogues available in the U.S. are exenatide (sold as Byetta) and liraglutide (sold as Victoza). They are sometimes referred to as GLP-1 receptor agonists. They are not considered first-choice drugs, but instead are typically used in combination with other drugs (except insulin).

Fun Fact for the diabetic version of Trivial Pursuit: Exenatide (Byetta) is a synthesized version of a protein initially discovered in the saliva of a lizard, the Gila monster.

How Do They Work?

It's complicated. First off, you need to know that a small intestine hormone, glucagon-like peptide-1 (GLP-1), is produced in response to a meal. This hormone increases insulin secretion by pancreas beta cells, suppresses glucagon after meals, inhibits emptying of the stomach, and inhibits appetite. Other effects are suppression of glucose production by the liver, and improved glucose uptake by tissues outside the liver. All this tends to lower blood sugar levels after meals.

The problem is that GLP-1 is quickly destroyed by an enzyme called DPP-4. We have available to us now chemicals similar to GLP-1, called GLP-1 analogues, that bind to the GLP-1 receptors and are resistant to degradation by the enzyme DPP-4. They essentially act like GLP-1, and they hang around longer.

GLP-1 levels, by the way, are decreased in type 2 diabetes.

The action of GLP-1 is dependent on blood sugar levels. If blood glucose is not elevated, GLP-1 doesn't go to work. From a practical viewpoint, this means that GLP-1-based therapies don't cause hypoglycemia.

We know little about long-term outcomes with these drugs, such as diabetic complications, health-related quality of life, or mortality.

Uses

Exenatide is FDA-approved for adults with type 2 diabetes who are not adequately controlled with metformin, sulfonylurea, or a thiazolidinedione (or a combination of these agents). So it's an add-on drug, not approved for use by itself. It's not approved for use with insulin therapy.

Liraglutide is FDA-approved for treatment of type 2 diabetes but is not recommended as initial therapy, although it does seem to be approved for use by itself. It has been used alone and also in combination with metformin, sulfonylurea, and/or thiazolidinediones. It's not approved for use with insulin therapy.

Dosing

They are available only as subcutaneous injections (under the skin). Exenatide is twice daily, starting at 5 mcg within 60 minutes prior to a meal. After four weeks, the dose is increased to 10 mcg twice daily.

Liraglutide is a once daily subcutaneous injection starting at 0.6 mg, increasing to 1.2 mg after one week. It is given without regard to meals. Maximum dose is 1.8 mg/day.

Side Effects

GLP-1 analogues tend to cause nausea, vomiting, and diarrhea in as many as four in 10 users. The nausea typically improves over time. They tend to cause weight loss. Both drugs might cause pancreatitis, which is potentially life-threatening. When used with a sulfonlyurea, hypoglycemia may occur.

Liraglutide might cause thyroid cancer. No risk of hypoglycemia when used as the sole diabetes drug.

Don't Use If You Have . . .

. . . severe kidney impairment (exenatide), Multiple Endocrine Neoplasia syndrome (liraglutide), or family history of medullary thyroid cancer (liraglutide).

Use GLP-1 analogues with caution if you have a history of pancreatitis or gastroparesis.

Use liraglutide with caution in patients with kidney or liver impairment.

41

INSULINS

Insulin is life-saving for type 1 diabetics. Many type 2 diabetics will eventually, if not at the outset, need to take insulin for adequate control of blood sugars, which should help prevent diabetes complications. My comments here are focused on various insulins as used by type 2 diabetics.

How Does Insulin Work?

Insulin is made by the pancreas to keep blood sugars from rising above a fairly strict range: 70–140 mg/dl or 3.89–7.78 mmol/l. [It has many other actions that I won't bother to reiterate here.] When we eat a meal containing carbohydrates (and proteins to a lesser extent), blood sugar starts to rise as we digest the carbs. Insulin drives the sugar into our body's cells for use as immediate energy or conversion to fat or glycogen as stored energy. About half of the daily insulin produced by a healthy body is "basal," meaning it's secreted into the bloodstream in a steady, low-volume amount, to keep the liver from making too much blood sugar (glucose), and for controlling fasting sugar levels. The other half is secreted in to the bloodstream in response to meals.

In type 2 diabetes, the body's tissues, at first, are resistant to the effect of insulin. So the pancreas has to secrete more than usual (hyperinsulinism). As the illness progresses, the pancreas cannot keep up with demand for more insulin and starts to "burn out," producing less insulin. As the burn out process continues, many diabetics need to start insulin injections. [These are generalities; there are exceptions.]

Types of Insulin

We could break them down into two types: human (identical in structure to human insulin) and analogs (minor molecular modifications to the usual human insulin molecule). The two human insulins are NPH and "regular." All the others are analogs. But most people don't care about that.

It's more helpful to distinguish insulins by the timing of their action:

Rapid Acting: lispro (e.g., Lantus), aspart (e.g., Novolog), glulisine (e.g., Apidra)

Short Acting: regular (e.g., Novolin R, Humulin R)

Intermediate to Long Acting: NPH, glargine (e.g., Lantus), determir (e.g., Levemir), NPL (neutral protamine lispro)

Rapid-acting insulins have an onset of action between 5 and 15 minutes, peak effect in 30 to 90 minutes, and duration of action of 2 to 4 hours.

Short-acting "regular insulin" has onset in 30 minutes, peaks in 2 to 4 hours, and works for 5 to 8 hours.

Intermediate to long-acting insulins start working in 2 hours, don't have a well-defined peak of action, and keep working for 20 or more hours (glargine) or for 6 to 24 hours (detemir).

All these times are gross approximations. Once the insulin is injected into the fat below the skin, it has to be absorbed into the bloodstream and transported to the tissues where it does its magic. Lots of factors affect this process. For instance, the thicker the fat tissue at the injection site, the slower the absorption. Absorption tends to be faster from the abdominal wall, slower from the arms, even slower from the thighs or buttocks. Absorption can vary from day to day in an individual even when injection site and technique are identical.

As you might have guessed, the short- and rapid-acting insulins are usually injected before a meal in anticipation of blood sugar rising as food is digested. The intermediate- and long-acting insulins imitate the healthy body's "basal" insulin.

Manufacturers also supply premixed insulins, combining intermediate or long-acting insulin with a short- or rapid-acting insulin. Examples are Humalog 75/25, Humulin 70/30, and Novolog 70/30.

In case you're wondering, modern insulin injections are barely painful, if at all.

Dose and Selection of Insulin

Anyone taking insulin must work closely with a physician or diabetes nurse educator on proper dosing, injection technique, and recognition and management of hypoglycemia (low blood sugar). Many type 2 diabetics get started just with an intermediate or long-acting insulin once or twice daily, with or without diabetes drugs by mouth. If and when the illness progresses, rapid-acting insulin may be added later.

Side Effects

By far the most common and worrisome is hypoglycemia.

MEGLITINIDES

Meglitinides—also called glinides—increase the output of insulin by the pancreas beta cells into the bloodstream. In that respect they are similar to sulfonylurea drugs, so the two classes are sometimes lumped together as insulin secretagogues. If the pancreas produces no insulin at all—as in most cases of type 1 diabetes—these drugs won't work.

Two meglitinides are available in the U.S.: repaglinide is sold as Prandin, and nateglinide as Starlix.

Meglitinides have about the same effectiveness as sulfonylureas, but are considerably more expensive. Repaglinide and nateglinide increase insulin secretion by the pancreas, working faster than sulfonylureas. They don't last as long as sulfonylureas, which may help avoid hypoglycemia. Glinides work mostly to reduce sugar levels after meals.

We don't know if these drugs affect death rates.

Uses

May be used alone or in combination with certain other diabetic drugs. Since they have the same mechanism of action, sulfonylureas and meglitinides would not normally be used together. In combination therapy, you want to use drug classes that work by different mechanisms.

Dosing

Starting dose for repaglinide is 0.5 mg by mouth before each meal. Maximum dose is 4 mg before each meal.

Nateglinide: 120 mg by mouth immediately before each meal.

45

Side Effects

Hypoglycemia is the most common and potentially serious adverse effect of the meglitinides, but may be less common than with sulfonylureas.

Weight gain is common.

Precautions . . .

Nateglinide: Use with great caution, if at all, in the setting of severe kidney disease and moderate to severe liver disease.

Repaglinide: Use cautiously in severe kidney and liver disease.

METFORMIN

Metformin is a major drug for treatment of type 2 diabetes. In fact, it's usually the first choice when a drug is needed.

Class

Biquanide (it's the only one in this class).

How Does It Work?

In short, metformin decreases glucose output by the liver. The liver produces glucose (sugar) either by breaking down glycogen stored there or by manufacturing glucose from smaller molecules and atoms. The liver then kicks the glucose into the bloodstream for use by other tissues. Insulin inhibits this function of the liver, thereby keeping blood sugar levels from getting too high. Metformin improves the effectiveness of insulin in suppressing sugar production. In other words, it works primarily by decreasing the liver's production of glucose.

Physicians talk about metformin as an "insulin sensitizer," primarily in the liver but also to a lesser extent in peripheral tissues such as fat tissue and muscle. It doesn't work without insulin in the body.

Metformin typically lowers fasting blood sugar by about 20% and hemoglobin A1c by 1.5% (absolute decrease, not relative).

When used as the sole diabetic medication, metformin is associated with decreased risk of death and heart attack, compared to therapy with sulfonylureas, thiazolidinediones, alpha-glucosidase inhibitors, and meglitinides.

Not uncommonly, metformin leads to a bit of weight loss and improved cholesterol levels. Insulin and sulfonylurea therapy, on the other hand, typically lead to weight gain of 8–10 pounds (4 kg) on average.

Usage

Metformin works by itself, but can also be used in combination with most of the other diabetic medications. It's usually taken 2–3 times daily.

Dose

Starting dose is typically 500 mg taken with the evening meal. The dose can be increased every week or two. If more than 500 mg/day is needed, the second dose—500 mg—is usually given with breakfast. Usual effective maximum dose is around 2,000 mg daily.

Side Effects

Metallic taste, diarrhea, belly pain, loss of appetite. Possible impaired absorption of vitamin B12, leading to anemia. When used alone, it has very little risk of hypoglycemia. Rare: lactic acidosis.

Don't Use Metformin If You Have . . .

Impaired kidney function, congestive heart failure of a degree that requires drug therapy (this is debatable), active liver disease, or chronic alcohol abuse.

PRAMLINTIDE

Pramlintide is sold in the U.S. as Symlin. It's only used in patients already taking meal-time rapid-acting insulin. Pramlintide may have a role in treatment of overweight type 2 diabetics inadequately controlled on insulin, or who experience weight gain refractory to diet and exercise.

Class

Amylin analogue.

How Does It Work?

Amylin is a hormone stored in pancreas beta cells and is secreted along with insulin. It affects glucose levels by several mechanisms, including slowed stomach emptying, regulation of glucagon secretion after meals, and by reducing food intake. Amylin and insulin levels rise and fall together, working jointly to control blood sugar levels. Amylin is relatively deficient in many cases of type 2 diabetes.

Pramlintide is a chemical similar in structure to amylin and causes similar effects. It allows insulin therapy to more easily match the body's needs in the after-meal period. It also promotes modest weight loss in obese patients.

Pramlintide therapy reduces hemoglobin A1c by 0.5 to 1% (absolute decrease, not relative).

We have no data on long-term health outcomes with this drug.

Uses

Pramlintide is FDA-approved for use in both type 1 diabetes and insulin-requiring type 2 diabetes. It can be used with metformin and/or sulfonylureas as long as insulin is also part of the regimen. It's probably best not to use it with exenatide and other GLP-1-based therapies.

Dosing

It's injected subcutaneously just before meals, starting with 60 mcg in type 2 diabetics. To avoid hypoglycemia at the start of treatment, the pre-meal rapid-acting injected insulin dose is usually reduced by half. Pramlintide should only be administered before meals that contain at least 30 grams of carbohydrate or 250 calories. The maximum dose is 120 mcg with each meal.

Side Effects

Nausea is the most common side effect but clears up in a few weeks. Pramlintide by itself does not cause hypoglycemia, but since it is always used with injectable insulin, hypoglycemia may occur—usually within three hours.

Don't Use If You Have . . .

. . . gastroparesis or hypoglycemia unawareness.

SULFONYLUREAS

Sulfonylureas (SUs) in 2011 are still the most widely used drugs for treatment of type 2 diabetes. At least six different SUs are in common usage in the U.S., including glipizide, glimiperide, and glyburide. They are often prescribed for patients who do not respond adequately to lifestyle modification and are intolerant of metformin, the usual first-choice drug.

Sulfonlylureas make the pancreas beta cells secrete more insulin into the bloodstream. The other drugs that do this are the meglitinides; these two classes are sometimes lumped together as insulin secretagogues. The sulfonylureas are less expensive.

This is a brief review pertinent to type 2 diabetes only—consult your physician or pharmacist for details. Remember that drug names vary by country and manufacturer.

How Do They Work?

Sulfonylureas increase the pancreas's production of insulin after a meal (second phase insulin secretion). If the pancreas beta cells are no longer producing any insulin, SUs won't work. SUs decrease fasting blood sugar by about 20% and hemoglobin A1c by 1 or 2% (absolute, not relative).

[Metiglinides have about the same effectiveness as SUs. Repaglinide and nateglinide increase the pancreas's output of insulin, working faster than sulfonylureas. They don't last as long as sulfonylureas, which may help avoid hypoglycemia. These two "glinides" work mostly to reduce sugar levels after meals.]

We don't know if SUs affect death rates.

Uses

May be used alone or in combination with certain other diabetic drugs. Since they have the same mechanism of action, sulfonylureas and meglitinides would not normally be used together. In combination therapy, you want to use drug classes that work by different mechanisms.

Dosing

SU dose depends on the particular one used. Some are taken by mouth once daily, others twice.

Side Effects

Hypoglycemia is the most severe adverse effect of the sulfonylureas. The duration of hypoglycemia seen with SUs is often much longer than you would predict by how much drug is in the bloodstream. Hypoglycemia is more common with the longer-acting drugs, such as glyburide and chlorpropamide. There is some concern that sulfonylureas are linked to poorer outcomes after a heart attack. SUs occasionally cause nausea, skin reactions, and elevations of liver function tests.

Weight gain is common.

When used with insulin or thiazolidinediones, these sulfonylurea adverse effects are more likely to appear: weight gain, fluid retention, congestive heart failure.

Precautions . . .

Consult your personal physician or pharmacist.

THIAZOLIDINEDIONES

Thiazolidinediones are more easily referred to as TZDs or glitazones. Compared to the usual first-choice drug for type 2 diabetes (metformin), the TZDs are significantly more expensive.

Remember that drug names—both generic and brand—may vary depending on country and manufacturer. In the U.S., rosiglitazone is sold as Avandia; pioglitazone as Actos.

How Do They Work?

In short, TZDs increase glucose utilization and decrease glucose production, leading to lower blood sugar levels. They sensitize several tissues to the effect of insulin. Insulin, among other actions, helps put circulating blood sugar into our muscles, fat cells, and (to a lesser extent) liver cells. So blood sugar levels fall. Thiazolidinediones make these tissues more sensitive to this effect of insulin. Insulin also suppresses glucose production by the liver, an effect enhanced by TZDs. They reduce insulin resistance.

TZDs may also help preserve pancreas beta cell function. Beta cells produce insulin.

They reduce both fasting and after-meal glucose levels. Fasting blood sugar drops and average of 40 mg/dl. Hemoglobin A1c falls by 1 to 1.5% (absolute, not relative).

TZDs tend to improve blood lipids: lower triglycerides, higher HDL cholesterol, decreased small, dense LDL cholesterol. Pioglitazone has the more pronounced effect.

They may help preserve pancreas beta cell function.

On a cellular level, they activate peroxisome proliferator-activated receptor-gamma, so they are sometimes referred to as PPAR-gamma agonists. Pioglitazone also affects PPAR-alpha.

Uses

TZDs can be used alone or in combination with insulin, metformin, and sulfonylureas in people with type 2 diabetes.

Dosing

Note that onset of action is delayed by several weeks, perhaps as many as 8–12 weeks.

Pioglitazone: Start at 15–30 mg/day by mouth. Maximum dose is 45 mg/day.

Rosiglitizone: Start at 4 mg/day by mouth. After 8–12 weeks, dose may be increased to 8 mg/day.

Side Effects

Weight gain is fairly common, through both fluid retention and increase in fat tissue. Weight gain with pioglitazone, for example, is around 6–12 pounds (3–5 kg). Mild anemia and puffy feet and hands (edema from fluid retention) are also seen. Fluid retention may ultimately cause congestive heart failure. This drug-induced fluid retention does not respond very well to fluid pills (diuretics).

The combination of insulin injections and TZD may increase the risk of heart failure.

Some studies suggest that rosiglitazone (Avandia) increases the risk of coronary heart disease, stroke, heart failure, and premature death, but other studies find no such effect. Nevertheless, many physicians prefer rosiglitazone's competitor, pioglitazone (Actos).

TZDs are associated with increased risk for broken bones, perhaps doubling the risk.

Macular edema—manifested by blurry vision—may occur infrequently.

When used as the sole diabetic medication, TZDs do not cause hypoglycemia. But when used with insulin injections or insulin secretagogues, low blood sugar can occur.

Don't Use If You . . .

. . . have a significant degree of congestive heart failure or active liver disease. Even a history of heart failure may be a reason to avoid TZDs. TZDs should probably not be used in women with low bone density or anyone else prone to fractures.

Don't use rosiglitazone if you can control blood sugars with other diabetes drugs, such as pioglitazone. The problem is that rosiglitazone seems to increases the risk of heart attack, heart failure, and death.

4

Hypoglycemia

Low-carbohydrate diets are often so effective at controlling blood sugars that low blood sugar becomes a serious risk for some diabetics. It's rarely a problem for prediabetics. But people with diabetes using particular drugs could develop life-threatening hypoglycemia, particularly when switching to a reduced-calorie or low-carb style of eating.

CARBOHYDRATES AND BLOOD SUGAR

Never forget that carbohydrate consumption has a major effect on blood sugar (glucose) levels—often causing a rise—in many people with type 2 diabetes and prediabetes. Most folks with diabetes are taking medications to lower their glucose levels.

Remember that the main components of food—called macronutrients—are proteins, fats, and carbohydrates. Common carbohydrate sources are:

- grains
- fruits
- starchy vegetables (e.g., potatoes, corn, peas, beans)
- milk products
- candy
- sweetened beverages
- other added sugars (e.g., table sugar, high fructose corn syrup, honey)

Low-carb and very-low-carb diets restrict the dieter's carbohydrate consumption rather dramatically. The standard American diet, for instance, provides 250–300 grams of carbohydrate daily, or 50-60% of total energy (calories). A low-carb diet may provide in the range of 50–130 grams daily, or 10 to 25% of total calories. A very-low-carb diet provides under 50 grams of carb daily (under 10% of all calories), often starting at 20–30 grams. With very-low-carb diets, our bodies must use fats instead of carbohydrates as an energy source, and a result of this fat metabolism is the generation of ketone bodies in the bloodstream. So very-low-carb diets are often called ketogenic diets.

Many dietitians have been taught that you must eat at least 130 grams of carbohydrate daily to provide a rich, readily available source of energy—glucose, specifically—to your brain in particular, and other tissues. Millions of "low-carbers"—people with a low-carb way of eating—know that isn't right, having proven it to themselves by experience. I personally lived on 30 grams (or less) daily for four months without problems with my brain or other organs. (Well, my wife might argue about the brain issue.) I felt fine and had plenty of energy.

In healthy people, prediabetics, and mild diabetics *not treated with medication*, carbohydrate restriction rarely causes low blood sugar problems (hypoglycemia). But in other diabetics, carbohydrate restriction can lead to serious, even life-threatening, symptoms of hypoglycemia.

DRUGS, DIET, AND HYPOGLYCEMIA

Traditional balanced diets for diabetics typically provide 50 to 60% of all calories as carbohydrates. Low-carb diets, remember, provide 25% or less of calories as carbohydrates. A diabetic trying to lose excess weight with a traditional balanced diet is told also to reduce total calories, which necessarily means lowering carbohydrate grams. So, hypoglycemia (low blood sugar) is also a potential problem for diabetics on these traditional reduced-calorie diets if they are taking particular diabetic medications.

Hypoglycemia, however, is an even greater risk for diabetics taking certain diabetic drugs while on a low-carb or very-low-carb diet. Serious, even life-threatening, symptoms of hypoglycemia may arise.

For diabetics taking certain diabetic drugs, carbohydrate restriction can lead to serious, even life-threatening, symptoms of hypoglycemia.

I hope I've made my point. This is dangerous territory. See the last chapter for names of drugs that can cause hypoglycemia.

HYPOGLYCEMIA: RECOGNITION AND MANAGEMENT

Hypoglycemia is the biggest immediate risk for a diabetic on drugs starting a carbohydrate-restricted diet. Traditional calorie-restricted diets also have the potential to cause hypoglycemia. Hypoglycemia means an abnormally low blood sugar (under 60–70 mg/dl or 3.33–3.89 mmol/l) associated with symptoms such as weakness, malaise, anxiety, irritability, shaking, sweating, hunger, fast heart rate, blurry vision, difficulty concentrating, or dizziness. Symptoms often start suddenly and without obvious explanation. If not recognized and treated, hypoglycemia can lead to incoordination, altered mental status (fuzzy thinking, disorientation, confusion, odd behavior, lethargy), loss of consciousness, seizures, and even death (rare).

You can imagine the consequences if you develop fuzzy thinking or lose consciousness while driving a car, operating dangerous machinery, or scuba diving.

Your personal physician and other healthcare team members will teach you how to recognize and manage hypoglycemia. Immediate early stage treatment involves ingestion of glucose as the preferred treatment—15 to 20 grams. You can get glucose tablets or paste at your local pharmacy without a prescription. Other carbohydrates will also work: six fl oz (180 ml) sweetened fruit juice, 12 fl oz (360 ml) milk, four tsp (20 ml) table sugar mixed in water, four fl oz (120 ml) soda pop, candy, etc. Fifteen to 30 grams of glucose or other carbohydrate should do the trick. Hypoglycemic symptoms respond within 20 minutes.

If level of consciousness is diminished such that the person cannot safely swallow, he will need a glucagon injection. Non-medical people can be trained to give the injection under the skin or into a muscle. Ask your doctor if you are at risk for severe hypoglycemia. If so, ask him for a prescription so you can get an emergency glucagon kit from a pharmacy.

Some people with diabetes, particularly after having the condition for many years, lose the ability to detect hypoglycemia just by the way they feel. This "hypoglycemia unawareness" is obviously more dangerous than being able to detect and treat hypoglycemia early on. Blood sugar levels may continue to fall and reach a life-threatening degree. Hypoglycemia unawareness can be caused by impairment of the nervous system (autonomic neuropathy) or by beta blocker drugs prescribed for high blood pressure or heart disease. People with hypoglycemia unawareness need to check blood sugars more frequently, particularly if driving a car or operating dangerous machinery.

Do not assume your sugar is low every time you feel a little hungry, weak, or anxious. Use your home glucose monitor for confirmation when able.

If you do experience hypoglycemia, discuss management options with your doctor: downward medication adjustment, shifting meal quantities or times, adjustment of exercise routine, eating more carbohydrates, etc. If you're trying to lose weight or control high blood sugars, reducing certain diabetic drugs makes more sense than eating more carbs. Eating at regular intervals three or four times daily may help prevent hypoglycemia. Spreading carbohydrate consumption evenly throughout the day may help. Someone most active during daylight hours as opposed to nighttime will generally do better eating carbs at breakfast and lunch rather than concentrating them at bedtime.

DRUG ADJUSTMENTS TO AVOID HYPOGLYCEMIA

Diabetics considering or following a low-carb or very-low-carb ketogenic diet must work closely with their personal physician and dietitian, especially to avoid hypoglycemia caused by certain classes of diabetic drugs. People who don't know the class of their diabetic medication should ask their physician or pharmacist. See the last chapter for names of diabetic drugs and classes that may cause hypoglycemia.

Clinical experience with thousands of patients has led to generally accepted guidelines that help avoid hypoglycemia in diabetics on medications.

Diabetics and prediabetics not being treated with pills or insulin rarely need to worry about hypoglycemia.

Similarly, diabetics treated only with diet, metformin, colesevalam, and/or an alpha-glucosidase inhibitor (acarbose, miglitol) should not have much, if any, trouble with hypoglycemia. The DPP4-inhibitors (sitagliptan and saxagliptin) do not seem to cause low glucose levels, whether used alone or combined with metformin or a thiazoladinedione.

Thiazolidinediones by themselves cause hypoglycemia in only 1 to 3% of users, but might cause a higher percentage in people on a reduced calorie diet. Bromocriptine may slightly increase the risk of hypoglycemia.

THESE DRUGS MAY CAUSE HYPOGLYCEMIA

Type 2 diabetics are at risk for hypoglycemia if they use the following drug classes. Also listed are a few of the individual drugs in some classes:

- insulin
- sulfonylureas: glipizide, glyburide, glimiperide, chlorpropamide, acetohexamide, tolbutamide
- meglitinides: repaglinide, nateglinide
- pramlintide plus insulin
- exenatide plus sulfonylurea
- possibly thiazolidinediones: pioglitazone, rosiglitazone
- possibly bromocriptine

Remember, drugs have both generic and brand names. The names vary from country to country, as well as by manufacturer. If you have any doubt about whether your diabetic drug has the potential to cause hypoglycemia, ask your physician or pharmacist.

MANAGEMENT STRATEGIES TO AVOID HYPOGLYCEMIA

Common management strategies for diabetics on the preceding drugs and starting a very-low-carb diet include:

- reduce the insulin dose by half
- change short-acting insulin to long-acting (such as glargine)
- stop the sulfonylurea, or reduce dose by half
- reduce the thiazolidinedione by half
- stop the meglitinide, or reduce the dose by half
- monitor blood sugars frequently, such as four times daily, at least until a stable pattern is established

- spread what few carbohydrates are eaten evenly throughout the day

Management also includes frequent monitoring of glucose levels with a home glucose monitor, often four to six times daily. Common measurement times are before meals and at bedtime. It may be helpful to occasionally wake at 3 AM and check a sugar level. To see the effect of a particular food or meal on glucose level, check it one or two hours after eating. Keep a record. When eating patterns are stable, and blood sugar levels are reasonable and stable, monitoring can be done less often. When food consumption or exercise habits change significantly, check sugar levels more often.

If you're thinking that many type 2 diabetics on low-carb and very-low-carb ketogenic diets use fewer diabetic medications, you're right. That's probably a good thing since the long-term side effects of many of the drugs we use are unknown. Remember Rezulin (troglitazone)? Introduced in 1997, it was pulled off the U.S. market in 2001 because of fatal liver toxicity.

5

Ketogenic Mediterranean Diet

INTRODUCTION

In 1797, Dr. John Rollo (a surgeon in the British Royal Artillery) published a book entitled *An Account of Two Cases of the Diabetes Mellitus.* He discussed his experience treating a diabetic Army officer, Captain Meredith, with a high-fat, high-meat, low-carbohydrate diet. Mind you, this was an era devoid of effective drug therapies for diabetes.

The soldier apparently had type 2 diabetes rather than type 1.

Rollo's diet led to loss of excess weight (original weight 232 pounds or 105 kg), elimination of symptoms such as frequent urination, and reversal of elevated blood and urine sugars.

This makes Dr. Rollo the original low-carb diabetic diet doctor. Many of the leading proponents of low-carb eating over the last two centuries—whether for diabetes or weight loss—have been physicians.

I've assembled a very-low-carbohydrate Ketogenic Mediterranean Diet specifically for people who have one or more of the following conditions:

- type 2 diabetes
- prediabetes
- metabolic syndrome
- excess body weight they want to lose with a low-carb Mediterranean-style diet

The Low-Carb Mediterranean diet builds on this foundation and is outlined in chapter six.

Diabetes and prediabetes always involve impaired carbohydrate metabolism: ingested carbs are not handled by the body in a healthy fashion, leading to high blood sugars and, eventually, poisonous complications.

"Metabolic syndrome" may be a new term for you. It's a constellation of clinical factors that are associated with increased future risk of type 2 diabetes and atherosclerotic complications such as heart attack and stroke. One in six Americans has metabolic syndrome. Diagnosis requires at least three of the following five conditions:

- high blood pressure (130/85 or higher, or using a high blood pressure medication)
- low HDL cholesterol: under 40 mg/dl (1.03 mmol/l) in a man, under 50 mg/dl (1.28 mmol/l) in a women (or either sex taking a cholesterol-lowering drug)

- triglycerides over 150 mg/dl (1.70 mmol/l) (or taking a cholesterol-lowering drug)
- abdominal fat: waist circumference 40 inches (102 cm) or greater in a man, 35 inches (89 cm) or greater in a woman
- fasting blood glucose over 100 mg/dl (5.55 mmol/l)

Metabolic syndrome and simple excess weight often involve impaired carbohydrate metabolism. Over time, excessive carbohydrate consumption can turn overweight and metabolic syndrome into predia- betes, then type 2 diabetes.

The key feature of the Ketogenic and Low-Carb Me- diterranean Diets is carbohydrate restriction, which directly addresses impaired carbohydrate metabol- ism naturally.

My primary goal with this program—the world's first low-carb Mediterranean diet—is to reap the health benefits of Mediterranean-style eating without los- ing control of blood sugars in people with diabetes and prediabetes. My secondary goal is loss of excess fat weight, if needed.

The American Diabetes Association recommends weight loss for all overweight diabetics. Its 2011 guidelines suggest three possible diets: "For weight loss, either low-carbohydrate [under 130 g/day], low-fat calorie-restricted, or Mediterranean diets may be effective in the short-term (up to two years)." My program gives you two out of three.

WHY "KETOGENIC"?

Your body gets nearly all its energy either from fats, or from carbohydrates like glucose and glycogen. In people eating normally, 60% of their energy at rest comes from fats. In a ketogenic diet, the carbohydrate content of the diet is so low that the body has to break down even more of its fat to supply energy needed by most tissues. Fat breakdown generates ketone bodies in the bloodstream. Hence, "ketogenic diet." Also called "very-low-carb diets," ketogenic diets have been around for over a hundred years.

Ketogenic diets have several practical advantages over other diets (disputed by some authorities):

- simplicity
- almost unlimited access to many high-protein and fatty foods
- less trouble with hunger
- better short-term weight loss than many other diets (long-term, too?)
- lower blood sugar levels, which is important to people with diabetes, prediabetes, and metabolic syndrome
- reduced insulin levels in people who often have elevated levels (hyperinsulinemia), which may help reduce chronic diseases like type 2 diabetes, high blood pressure, some cancers, and coronary heart disease
- higher levels of HDL cholesterol and lower triglycerides, which may reduce risk of heart disease
- it obviously works well for a significant portion of the overweight population, but not for everybody
- better adherence to the program compared with other diets, at least for the short-term

WHY "MEDITERRANEAN"?

For years, the Mediterranean diet has been widely recognized as the healthiest diet for the general population. The enduring popularity of the Mediterranean diet is attributable to three things:

1. Taste
2. Variety
3. Health benefits

(In this context, I'm using "diet" to refer to the usual food and drink of a person, not a weight-loss program.)

The scientist most responsible for the popularity of the diet, Ancel Keys, thought the heart-healthy aspects of the diet were related to low saturated fat consumption. He also thought the lower blood cholesterol levels in Mediterranean populations (at least Italy and Greece) had something to do with it, too. Dietary saturated fat does tend to raise cholesterol levels.

Even if Keys was wrong about saturated fat and cholesterol levels being positively associated with heart disease, numerous studies (involving eight countries on three continents) indicate that the Mediterranean diet is one of the healthiest around. (See the Annotated Bibliography for the most recent studies.)

Strong evidence supports the Mediterranean diet's association with:

- increased lifespan
- lower rates of cardiovascular disease such as heart attacks and strokes
- lower rates of cancer (prostate, breast, uterus,

colon)
- lower rates of dementia
- lower incidence of type 2 diabetes

Weaker supporting evidence links the Mediterranean diet with:

- slowed progression of dementia
- prevention of melanoma (serious skin cancer)
- lower severity of type 2 diabetes, as judged by diabetic drug usage and fasting blood sugars
- less risk of developing obesity
- better blood pressure control in the elderly
- improved weight loss and weight control in type 2 diabetics
- improved control of asthma
- reduced risk of developing diabetes after a heart attack
- reduced risk of mild cognitive impairment
- prolonged life of Alzheimer disease patients
- lower rates and severity of chronic obstructive pulmonary disease
- lower risk of gastric (stomach) cancer
- less risk of macular degeneration
- less Parkinsons disease
- increased chance of pregnancy in women undergoing fertility treatment
- reduced prevalence of metabolic syndrome (when supplemented with nuts)
- lower incidence of asthma and allergy-like symptoms in children of women who followed the Mediterranean diet while pregnant

So what exactly is this traditional, healthy "Mediterranean diet"? Here are the predominant features:

- it maximizes natural whole foods and minimizes highly processed ones
- small amounts of red meat

- less than four eggs per week
- low to moderate amounts of poultry and fish
- daily fresh fruit
- seasonal locally grown foods with minimal processing
- concentrated sugars only a few times per week
- wine in low to moderate amounts, and usually taken at mealtimes
- milk products (mainly cheese and yogurt) in low to moderate amounts
- olive oil as the predominant fat
- abundance of foods from plants: vegetables, fruits, beans, potatoes, nuts, seeds, breads and other whole grain products
- naturally low in saturated fat, trans fats, and cholesterol
- naturally high in fiber, phytonutrients, vitamins (e.g., folate), antioxidants, and minerals (especially when compared with concentrated, refined starches and sugars in a modern Western diet)
- naturally high in monounsaturated and polyunsaturated fats, particularly as a replacement for saturated fats

WHAT'S WRONG WITH PURE MEDITERRANEAN?

The Mediterranean diet poses a problem for people with diabetes and prediabetes. It's relatively high in carbohydrates, which tend to raise blood sugars too high. The result could be diabetic complications or the need for more and more diabetic medications with unknown long-term side effects.

Despite an emphasis on carb-rich bread, pasta, fruits, legumes, and certain vegetables, the Mediterranean diet has several healthy components compatible with a very-low-carb eating style:

- olive oil
- nuts and seeds
- wine
- fish
- cheese
- Mediterranean spices

POTENTIAL PROBLEMS WITH VERY-LOW-CARB EATING

Long-term effects of a very-low-carb or ketogenic diet in most people are unclear—they may have better or worse overall health—we just don't know for sure yet. Perhaps some people gain a clear benefit, while others—with different metabolisms and genetic make-up—are worse off.

If the diet results in major weight loss that lasts, we may see longer lifespan, less type 2 diabetes, less cancer, less heart disease, less high blood pressure, and fewer of the other obesity-related medical conditions.

Ketogenic diets are generally higher in protein, total fat, saturated fat, and cholesterol than some other diets. Some authorities are concerned this may increase the risk of coronary heart disease and stroke; the latest evidence indicates otherwise (see Annotated Bibliography).

Some authorities worry that ketogenic diets have the potential to cause kidney stones, osteoporosis (thin, brittle bones), gout, deficiency of vitamins and minerals, and may worsen existing kidney disease. Others disagree.

It's clear that compliance with very-low-carb diets is difficult to maintain for six to 12 months. Many folks can't do it for more than a couple weeks. Potential long-term effects, therefore, haven't come into play for most users. When used for weight loss, regain of lost weight is a problem (but regain is a major issue with all weight-loss programs). I anticipate that the majority of non-diabetics who try a ketogenic diet will stay on it for only one to six months. After that, more carbohydrates can be added to gain the potential long-term benefits of additional fruits and vegetables, legumes, and whole grains.

Or not.

People with type 2 diabetes or prediabetes may be so pleased with the metabolic effects of the ketogenic diet that they'll stay on it long-term.

CARBOHYDRATE INTOLERANCE

Diabetics and prediabetics—plus many folks with metabolic syndrome—must remember that their bodies do not, and cannot, handle dietary carbs in a normal, healthy fashion. In a way, carbs are toxic to them. Toxicity may lead to amputations, blindness, kidney failure, nerve damage, poor circulation, frequent infections, premature heart attacks and death, among other things.

Diabetics and prediabetics simply don't tolerate carbs in the diet like other people. If you don't tolerate something, you have to give it up, or at least cut way back on it. Lactose-intolerant individuals give up milk and other lactose sources. Celiac disease patients don't tolerate gluten, so they give up wheat and other sources of gluten. One of every five high blood pressure patients can't handle normal levels of salt in the diet; they have to cut back or their pressure's too high. Patients with phenylketonuria don't tolerate phenylalanine and have to restrict foods that contain it. If you're allergic to penicillin, you have to give it up. If you don't tolerate carbs, you have to give them up or cut way back. I'm sorry.

PRECAUTIONS AND DISCLAIMER

The ideas and suggestions in this document are provided as general educational information only and should not be construed as medical advice or care. Information herein is meant to complement, not replace, any advice or information from your personal health professional. All matters regarding your health require supervision by a personal physician or other appropriate health professional familiar with your current health status. Always consult your personal physician before making any dietary or exercise changes. Steve Parker, M.D., and the publisher disclaim any liability or warranties of any kind arising directly or indirectly from use of this diet. If any medical problems develop, always consult your personal physician. Only your physician can provide you medical advice. You should not follow this diet if you are a child, pregnant or lactating, have alcoholism or history of alcohol abuse, have abnormal liver or kidney function, or have gout or a high uric acid blood level. Your physician may have to adjust medication dosages—particularly blood pressure pills and diabetic drugs—if you follow this diet.

LET'S GET STARTED!

The Ketogenic Mediterranean Diet is a very-low-carb diet—20 to 40 grams of digestible carbohydrate daily—designed for control of high blood sugars and loss of excess body fat. "Digestible carbohydrate" is the total carbohydrate grams minus the fiber grams of carbohydrate that you can't digest and utilize as an energy source.

For you nutrition science geeks, here's the macronutrient breakdown. Of the total calories eaten, 7–10% are from carbohydrate, 55–65% are from fat, 22–30% are from protein, and 5–10% are from alcohol.

You'll find a three-page printable version of the basic Ketogenic Mediterranean Diet (KMD) here: http://advancedmediterraneandiet.com/printabledocuments.html.

HERE'S WHAT YOU'LL EAT:

1) Unlimited fish, meat, chicken, turkey, eggs, shrimp, lobster

2) Fish, at least 4 oz (115 g) daily

3) Olive oil, virgin or extra-virgin, at least 2–3 tbsp (30–45 ml) daily

4) Nuts and seeds, 1 oz (28 g) daily

5) Vegetables, up to 14 oz (400 g) daily

6) Wine, 6–12 fl oz (180–360 ml) daily (see alternatives in Miscellaneous Comments)

7) Cheese, up to 3 oz (85 g) daily, optional

8) Daily supplements:

   • 1 or 2 plain Centrum multivitamin/multimineral supplements (two if over

73

250 lb or 114 kg)
- Magnesium oxide 250 mg
- Calcium carbonate 500 mg elemental calcium (500 mg twice daily if over 250 lb or 114 kg)
- Extra vitamin D to reach total of 1,000–1,200 IU (each Centrum has 400 IU)
- Potassium gluconate 2,750 mg (450 mg elemental potassium) or Morton Salt Substitute (potassium chloride) ¼ tsp (1.2 g)
- If prone to constipation: sugar-free Metamucil powder 1–2 rounded tsp (5.8–11.6 g) in water
- At least three quarts or liters of water

What makes it Mediterranean? Natural whole foods, fish, olive oil, nuts, wine, cheese, spices.

What's not Mediterranean? Unlimited meat and animal proteins, and absence of most sweet fruits, high-carbohydrate vegetables, grains, legumes, pasta, honey, and yogurt. These may come later.

You can track your blood sugars and consumption of the major foods with the "KMD & LCMD Daily Log" available for free at http://advancedmediterraneandiet.com/printabledocuments.html

See chapter seven for "A Week of Meals" consistent with the Ketogenic Mediterranean Diet. Or just use your imagination while following the guidelines above.

WARNING

Wine and other alcoholic beverages are dangerous. You should not drink wine or any alcohol if you have a history of alcohol abuse or alcoholism, have liver or pancreas disease, are pregnant or trying to become pregnant, may have the need to operate dangerous equipment or machinery—such as driving a car—while under the influence of alcohol, or have demonstrated inability to limit yourself to acceptable intake levels.

FOOD CATEGORY COMMENTS:

1. Protein Group

This includes fish, meat, chicken, turkey, eggs, shrimp, lobster, and fried pork skins. Try to avoid overly processed protein products; aim for pure and simple. Processed meats may have added carbohydrates, nitrites, and other chemicals you don't need. Canned products are OK. *Eat until full or satisfied, not stuffed.*

2. Fish

Canned fish may be more affordable and convenient. Cold-water fatty fish have more omega-3 fatty acids: trout, salmon, sardines, mackerel, albacore/white tuna, herring, swordfish, halibut, sea bass. If you are pregnant, trying to become pregnant, or a nursing mother, avoid eating king mackerel, swordfish, shark, and tilefish (sold as golden snapper or golden bass); these fish may contain amounts of mercury harmful to breast-fed infants and babies in the womb. If you eat lots of locally caught freshwater fish, especially if you are a women of childbearing age, check with your regional governmental authorities regarding contaminants. In the U.S., the appropriate state agency is usually the Health Department or Game and Fish Department. Note that adult medical problems attributable to chemical fish contamination are exceedingly rare.

3. Olive oil

Use virgin or extra virgin oil in vinaigrette or other olive oil-based salad dressing. Sauté with it. Fry eggs and steak with it. Drink it straight if you want!

4. Nuts and Seeds

Almonds, walnuts, pecans, Brazil nuts, hazelnuts (filberts), macadamia nuts, peanuts (a legume), Spanish peanuts, pistachios, pine nuts, sunflower seeds, pumpkin seeds in shells. These average 3 g of digestible carbohydrate per ounce (28 g). Sunflower seeds, peanuts, and pistachios are the highest-carb: 3.5 to 4 g per ounce (28 g). Sorry, no cashews.

5. Vegetables & Fruit

(A) Raw salad vegetables: lettuce, mushrooms, radishes, spinach, alfalfa sprouts, cucumber, tomato, scallions, parsley, jicama, arugula, endive, radicchio, chard, sweet peppers, avocado, olives (pickled green or ripe black), pickles (dill or sour, not sweet or "bread and butter"). Average digestible carbohydrate per 7 oz serving (200 g) is 5 g. The highest digestible carb counts are in scallions and jicama (8 g), and sweet peppers (7g).

(B) Solid vegetables, often cooked: snow peas, broccoli, summer squash, tomato, onion, cauliflower, eggplant, Brussels sprouts, asparagus, okra, sauerkraut (canned), green beans. These average 8 g of digestible carbohydrate per 7 oz serving (200 g). Onion is highest at 14 g. Weigh these before cooking.

6. Wine

Red wine (e.g., Burgundy, Cabernet Sauvignon, or Merlot) may be healthier than white (e.g., Sauvignon blanc, Riesling, Pinot Grigio). One fl oz (30 ml) of wine has 1 g of carbohydrate.

7. Cheese

Real, regular cheese; not low-fat. Mozzarella, provolone, swiss, cheddar, blue, Monterey, Colby, brie, Parmesan, feta, gouda, ricotta, cottage. These have 1 g carbohydrate per oz (28 g). Other cheeses have too many carbs.

MISCELLANEOUS COMMENTS:

Alternatives to wine (choose only one daily):
- Extra 200 g (7 oz) vegetables, and consider a grape extract supplement daily, or
- 20 g (0.7 oz) of dark chocolate (65-85% cacao) daily, or
- Beer, 12 fl oz (360 ml) daily, but must have under 10 g of carbs, or
- Distilled spirits (whiskey, rum, vodka, gin), 80 proof, 1.5 fl oz (45 ml) daily

Additional daily optional oils, spices, and condiments (unlimited unless noted):

Butter, plant oils (strongly favor olive oil), vinegar (cider, red wine, or distilled), balsamic vinegar (2 tsp or 10 ml daily), salt, pepper, genuine mayonnaise (not low-fat), yellow mustard (1 tbsp or 15 ml daily), salad dressing (with three or fewer grams of carbohydrate per 2 tbsp or 30 ml) (2 tbsp daily), Worcestershire sauce (1 tbsp or 15 ml), A.1. Steak Sauce (1 tbsp or 15 ml)

Prominent Mediterranean spices: paprika, cumin, turmeric, cinnamon, ginger (0.35 oz or 10 g raw root, or 2 tsp or 10 ml ground spice daily), coriander, anise, Spanish saffron, lemon or lime juice (2 tbsp or 30 ml daily), mint, parsley, garlic (3 cloves daily), dill pepper, and sumac

Tea and coffee in moderation are fine. Don't add milk to them; use full-fat cream or high-fat half-and-half.

All of the recommended supplements are readily available at supermarkets and pharmacies at a reasonable cost.

I recommend Centrum for people on the Ketogenic Mediterranean Diet. Why Centrum? It's been around for years and has a good reputation. It's widely available at a reasonable price. A different brand of multivitamin/multimineral supplement may be fine if it's close to Centrum's components. Since the composition of plain Centrum could change at any time (or be concocted differently in non-U.S. countries), listed below are the contents of the U.S. product in 2011. Here are the component amounts with "% Daily Values" in parentheses:

Vitamin A 3,5000 IU (70%), Vitamin C 60 mg (100%), Vitamin D 400 IU (100%), Vitamin E 30 IU (100%), Vitamin K 25 mcg (31%), Thiamin 1.5 mg (100%), Riboflavin 1.7 mg (100%), Niacin 20 mg (100%), Vitamin B6 2 mg (100%), Folic Acid 400 mcg (100%), Vitamin B12 6 mcg (100%), Biotin 30 mcg (10%), Pantothenic Acid 10 mg (100%), Calcium 200 mg (20%), Iron 18 mg (100%), Phosphorus 20 mg (2%), Iodine 150 mcg (100%), Magnesium 50 mg (13%), Zinc 11 mg (73%), Selenium 55 mcg (79%), Copper 0.5 mg (25%), Manganese 2.3 mg (115%), Chromium 35 mcg (29%), Molybdenum 45 mcg (60%), Chloride 72 mg (2%), Potassium 80 mg (2%), Boron 75 mcg, Nickel 5 mcg, Silicon 2 mg, Tin 10 mcg, Vanadium 10 mcg.

U.S. government authorities recommend Percent Daily Values for average non-pregnant healthy adults eating 2,000 calorie a day.

Need a sweet, crunchy treat? Metamucil Fiber Wafers (12 g each), two per week.

Don't just eat the same eight or 10 items—aim for great variety. For meal ideas, see chapter seven for a week of meals and special recipes.

You'll be eating lots of salad.

You'll need a scale to measure your vegetables and to follow the optional recipes in chapter seven.

To make your food shopping easier, you can print a grocery shopping list of all foods on the Ketogenic and Low-Carb Mediterranean Diets when you visit this web page:
http://advancedmediterraneandiet.com/printabledocuments.html

WHAT COULD GO WRONG?

Very-low-carb ketogenic diets have been associated with headaches, bad breath, easy bruising, nausea, fatigue, aching, muscle cramps, constipation, and dizziness, among other symptoms. "Induction flu" may occur around days two through five, consisting of achiness, easy fatigue, and low energy. It clears up after a few days.

Very-low-carb ketogenic diets may have the potential to cause osteoporosis (thin, brittle bones), kidney stones, low blood pressure, constipation, gout, high uric acid in the blood, excessive loss of sodium and potassium in the urine, worsening of kidney disease, deficiency of calcium and vitamins A, B, C, and D, among other adverse effects.

Athletic individuals who perform vigorous exercise should expect a deterioration in performance levels during the first three to four weeks of any ketogenic very-low-carb diet. The body needs that time to adjust to burning mostly fat for fuel rather than carbohydrate.

Competitive weight-lifters or other anaerobic athletes (e.g., sprinters) will be hampered by the low muscle glycogen stores that accompany ketogenic diets. They need more carbohydrates.

WHAT'S NEXT?

I recommend that anyone trying the Ketogenic Mediterranean Diet give it a good eight to twelve weeks. Then evaluate whether it's time to move on to the Low-Carb Mediterranean Diet (with a bit more variety) discussed in the next chapter.

6

Low-Carb Mediterranean Diet

The foundation of the Low-Carb Mediterranean Diet is the Ketogenic Mediterranean Diet (KMD) covered in the last chapter. The Low-Carb Mediterranean Diet loosens up on food restrictions and introduces additional carbohydrates as long as glucose control and weight management don't deteriorate.

You could call the Ketogenic Mediterranean Diet a Conversion Phase because your body is switching to an energy metabolism based on fats and proteins instead of carbohydrates. Or we could call it a Watershed Phase since a watershed is "a critical point that marks a division or a change of course; a turning point."

Some may stay on the KMD long-term, so it's freestanding.

But others will move on to the Low-Carb Mediterranean Diet (LCMD), adding more energy and nutrients from plants while managing blood sugar levels and weight.

Eighty-five percent of people with type 2 diabetes carry excess weight. The Ketogenic and Low-Carb Mediterranean Diets will help with that issue. But just as importantly, they lower and smooth out the elevated blood sugars characteristic of diabetes and prediabetes, regardless of weight.

I will assume readers of this chapter have been following the Ketogenic Mediterranean Diet for at least a couple weeks, if not for several months or more. I recommend at least 8–12 weeks. Many followers—diabetic or not—wanted to lose some excess weight with a Mediterranean-style diet. Others, already at healthy weights, just wanted better control of blood sugars or metabolic syndrome.

At this point you're ready for a change either because you've reached your weight-loss goal or you want a greater variety of carbohydrates (carbs). Stay familiar with the KMD because it is the foundation for everything that will follow. You're not really done with it; you're adding to it, moving from a very-low-carb diet to a low-carb diet.

Perhaps you've been losing weight steadily with the KMD and are not yet at your goal weight but need more food variety. Many continue to lose excess weight with the Low-Carb Mediterranean Diet, although it tends to be easier with the KMD. If weight loss stalls, just return to the KMD.

Alternatively, you may be interested in eating more of the plant-based foods that may yield the documented health benefits of the traditional Mediterranean diet.

The KMD may be perfectly healthy long-term; we just don't know for sure. On the other hand, there is at least some evidence that additional carbohydrates, as in the Low-Carb Mediterranean Diet, may be even healthier. For example, some scientific studies link fruit and vegetable consumption with lower rates of cancer, stroke, and coronary heart disease. [Other studies find no benefit.] Whole grain consumption is associated with lower rates of cardiovascular disease, including heart attacks and strokes. Legumes (such as beans and peas) are a great source of fiber to counteract the constipation common with very-low-carb diets like the KMD. Fruits and vegetables as components of the Mediterranean diet may contribute to longevity.

And many carbohydrates just plain taste good!

Nearly all the studies linking fruits, vegetables, whole grains, and legumes with improved health were done in general populations, not specifically in diabetics. Whether diabetics and prediabetics benefit is not entirely clear. If such consumption raises blood sugar levels too much, then health outcomes will be worse.

My primary goal with this program is to reap the health benefits of a Mediterranean style diet without losing control of blood sugars in diabetics and prediabetics.

A quick reminder for readers who may have started this book on this chapter: low-carb eating has the potential to drop blood sugar levels dangerously low in people with diabetes who take certain medications to control blood sugar. If this applies to you,

you must work closely with your personal physician and review chapter five: Hypoglycemia.

In case you haven't noticed, I use "blood sugar" and "glucose level" interchangeably.

OVERVIEW OF THE LOW-CARB MEDITERRANEAN DIET

You've been eating 20 to 30 grams of carbohydrate daily on the KMD. Now you're going to increase to 40–100 grams daily, gradually adding carbs that may have beneficial effects on health and longevity. Adding excessive carbs will lead inevitably to regain of lost weight, a stall in weight-loss progress, or to elevated blood sugars.

Most people reading this have type 2 diabetes, pre-diabetes, or metabolic syndrome and have had trouble controlling their weight or blood sugar levels with their former ways of eating. A few readers are entirely new to the world of diabetes. In all these cases, we want to avoid adding carbohydrates that sabotage control of blood sugars and metabolic syndrome. That sabotage may take two forms:

- eating particular carbs that will spike your blood sugars too high and for too long, or
- excessive amounts of carbs, which will do the same

For non-diabetics and those with normal carbohydrate metabolism, carbs that potentially raise blood sugar too much are not an immediate issue. But even for non-diabetics, these glucose-producing foods are associated—at least in women—with excessive body weight, future diabetes, heart disease, and gallbladder disease. So we may as well avoid them.

If you are not at your goal weight already, adding too many carb grams now will impair your ability to convert your body fat into energy. Eat too many carbs, and your body will use them for the energy it needs rather than your body's fat. You may well continue to lose weight eating 40, 60, or 100 grams a day, but maybe not. Everybody is different. Many diabetics will not be able to handle over 70 grams of carb daily. Some, not even that much. Continue to weigh yourself daily. Diabetics must monitor their blood sugar levels as discussed elsewhere.

LET'S GET STARTED ON LCMD!

So, what healthy carbs are we going to add to the Ketogenic Mediterranean Diet, transforming it into the LCMD? Fruits, more vegetables (including starchy ones), legumes, yogurt and other dairy products, and whole grains.

To avoid carb overdose and loss of glucose control, we're adding back carbs incrementally and slowly.

I've divided the new carbohydrates into groups and specified a serving size for each source of carbs. Each serving has about 7.5 grams of digestible carbohydrate.

What you do next is add one daily carb serving from the list of Carb Groups and Serving Sizes (see end of chapter) and see what happens with your glucose levels—and weight if that's an issue—over the next week. This is not one carb serving on Monday, two on Tuesday, three on Wednesday, etc. It's seven new carb servings per week, one on each day.

Essentially, you still eat the Ketogenic Mediterranean Diet but are adding a daily carb serving. If your glucose levels rise significantly, you have unwanted weight gain, or your weight loss progress stalls, you've added too many carbs and must cut back, or try different carb sources. See chapter two for acceptable blood sugar levels.

On the other hand, if you handled the extra carb serving without trouble for a week, you may add one more daily carb serving. Monitor your progress for another week.

If you're handling those carbs, you may increase by one additional carb serving every week. You've added too much carb if your glucose levels rise too much, you gain unwanted weight, or your weight loss progress stalls. Then you must cut back or try different carbs—especially different carb groups.

Many people who have diabetes, prediabetes, or weight management problems will not be able to increase carbs to more than six additional daily servings. Either weight or blood sugars will rise to unacceptable levels. But that's OK because you don't necessarily need more carbs for a long and healthy life. For many folks, additional carbs are unhealthy.

Diabetics and prediabetics should probably distribute, eventually, their additional carbs evenly among two or three daily meals. Eating two or three new additional carb servings all at once as a bedtime snack, for example, is likely to cause high blood sugars through the night and into the next morning. On the other hand, those same carbs eaten at breakfast and followed by an exercise session an hour later might be handled just fine. Your home glucose monitor will be indispensible in this arena.

Many diabetics find that carbs eaten for breakfast tend to sabotage blood sugar control more so than carbs eaten later in the day. The only way to find out is to experiment.

By the way, if you wish to cut back on your animal protein consumption at this point, feel free. It's your choice. I'd continue to eat cold-water fatty fish at least two or three times weekly, along with the usual olive oil and nuts.

Are you with me so far?

WHICH CARBS TO ADD

OK, so you're going to add some carbs to your diet, but which ones? Again, I'm assuming at this point you have diabetes, prediabetes, or metabolic syndrome. For the potential health benefits, I'd add carbs in this order:

- fruits
- more vegetables
- legumes
- yogurt and other dairy products
- whole grains

This is just a loose guideline, not a commandment. I suggest everyone eventually add one or two servings of fruit daily, classic fruits rather than technical fruits like tomato and avocado already on the KMD. Legumes, yogurt and other dairy products are listed after fruits and veggies because the evidence in favor of their long-term health benefits is not as strong.

For people with normal carbohydrate metabolism, I'd list whole grains second or third rather than last, but in diabetics . . .

. . . grains are problematic. Diabetics are prone to developing blockages in their heart arteries that can cause heart attacks and premature death. Consumption of whole grains on a regular basis is associated with significantly lower risk of developing heart disease. But there's a fly in the ointment. Grains, even whole grain products, have a relatively high glycemic index, meaning they cause spikes in blood glucose which could have adverse long-term impact. Nearly all the studies linking whole grain consumption with less heart disease were done in the general population, not the diabetic population. Whole grains could be even healthier for diabetics than the general population—we just don't know.

Diabetics who see a significant spike in blood sugar after grain consumption could address that with higher dosages of diabetic medications. Would that be healthier than avoiding grains? As of 2011, we just don't know.

Eating grains with a meal containing fat and protein also tends to smooth out or eliminate blood sugar spikes. That goes for other high-glycemic-index carbs, too, like potatoes.

Yogurt deserves special mention because it's a component of the traditional doctor-recommended Mediterranean diet. It's a great source of calcium, a critical mineral for healthy bones, nerves, and muscles. Does it have anything special you couldn't get elsewhere? Probably not.

Now you're ready to enhance the KMD with an extra carb serving daily. Why not start with a fruit? Choose a variety of items within any given carb group, and try eventually to eat from multiple carb groups. Variety ensures you get adequate vitamins, minerals, and phytonutrients.

Nevertheless, just to be sure, continue your supplements as on the KMD. If you're sick of taking them, drop the calcium first, potassium second, then magnesium. Wait a couple weeks between each discontinuation, and monitor how you feel. Any weakness? Fatigue? Muscle cramps? Restart the dropped supplement and see if it resolves the issue.

Things are getting a little complicated now. If your glucose levels get out of control or you regain lost fat weight, you can always return to home base: the Ketogenic Mediterranean Diet.

CARB GROUPS & SERVING SIZES FOR THE DIABETIC MEDITERRANEAN DIET

[Each serving has about 7.5 grams of digestible carbohydrate.]

FRUITS

apple, a third of medium-sized one (54 g)
banana, one third (39 g)
peach, ½ of medium (75 g)
strawberry halves, two thirds of a cup (75 g)
blueberries, ½ cup (75 g)
raspberries, 1 cup (123 g)
blackberries, 1 cup (144 g)
cantaloupe, ½ cup cubes (80 g)
honeydew, 1 cup of cubes (85 g)
date, medjool, ½ date (12 g)

orange, navel, ½ (70 g)
pear, a third of medium-sized one (60 g)
pomegranate, ¼ of 4" (10 cm) diameter fruit (70g)
tangerine, ½ (44 g)
grapefruit, ½ (61 g)
cherries, sweet, raw, a third of a cup (45 g)
grapes, a third of a cup (50 g)
raisins, seedless, 20 (9 g)
nectarine, medium, ½ (70 g)
mango, slices, a third of a cup (55 g)
pineapple, raw chunks, a third of a cup (55g)
lime/lemon juice, raw, 2 limes or lemons (88 g)
watermelon, diced, two thirds of a cup (100 g)

VEGETABLES AND FRUITS

potato, white, raw, flesh and skin,
    ¼ of medium potato (53 g)
corn, canned, drained, ¼ cup (41g)
carrots, raw, strips or slices, ¾ cup (92 g)
sweet potato, raw, a third of 5 inch-long (13 cm)
    tater (45 g)
beets, canned, drained solids, ¾ cup slices (130 g)
peas, green, canned or frozen, ½ cup (67 g)
spaghetti squash, cooked, 1 cup (155 g)
KMD mixed veggies, 7 oz (200 g)

LEGUMES

peas, split, mature seeds, cooked/boiled,
    ¼ cup (49 g)
peas, black-eyed (cowpeas), canned, ¼ cup (60 g)
soybeans, mature seeds, roasted, 1.5 oz (42 g)
soybeans, mature seeds, cooked/boiled,
    1 cup (170 g)
beans, mature seeds, cooked/boiled, ¼ cup (43 g)
    (beans = black, kidney, navy, pinto, white, fava,
    chickpeas/garbanzo)

YOGURT AND MILK PRODUCTS

yogurt, plain whole milk, ½ cup
milk, whole, ½ cup
milk, 1% milk fat, ½ cup
Fage Greek, "total 2%", ½ cup (get full-fat version
    if available)
Voskos plain original Greek yogurt, ½ cup

GRAINS

bread, whole wheat, ½ slice (15 g)
bread, Ezekial 4:19, ½ slice
pasta, 100% whole grain, dry, 12 g
Ry-Krisp crackers, 4.5 x 2.5" (11 x 6 cm) (11 g)
Triscuit crackers x 3 (14 g)
cracker, whole wheat, 14 g
tortilla (Mission), 8" (20 cm) whole grain,
    a third of a tortilla (16 g)
oats, dry whole grain, a third of a cup uncooked
    (13 g)
oats, steel-cut, uncooked, 1.3 tbsp (13 g)
rice, brown, cooked, 3 tbsp
quinoa, cooked, 3 tbsp (35 g)
barley, pearled, cooked, 3 tbsp (30g)
shredded wheat, plain, sugar-free (11 g)
cereal, FiberOne, original, plain,
    a third of a cup or 5 tbsp (75 ml)
Kellogg's All-Bran original or
    All-Bran Bran Buds, ¼ cup (15 g)

FOR YOUR CONVENIENCE . . .

You can print most of this chapter and a grocery shopping list for the both the KMD and LCMD at this web page:

http://advancedmediterraneandiet.com/printabledo cuments.html

Welcome to the Low-Carb Mediterranean Diet!

7

A Week of Meals + Special Recipes

This chapter provides seven days of meals consistent with the Ketogenic Mediterranean Diet, the foundation of the Low-Carb Mediterranean diet. Even if you follow the guidelines and restrictions "to a T," the Ketogenic Mediterranean Diet provides lots of variety, limited mostly by your imagination. You're going to eat lots of natural, whole foods made by God, and few processed, man-made foods.

You don't even have to do any cooking if you don't want. Avoid cooking altogether by using canned fish and meats along with raw whole foods and commercially prepared nuts, cheese, olive oil, wine, and spices. But many will appreciate the added variety and tastes that cooking brings to the table.

AS SIMPLE AS YOU LIKE

When I was following the KMD myself, a typical day started with a breakfast of cooked eggs with or without bacon, sausage, pre-cooked microwaved bratwurst, or left-over steak or chicken. Lunch was a large salad tossed with both olive oil vinaigrette and canned tuna (or the salad/vinaigrette and a separate tin of sardines or kippered herring). If vinaigrette wasn't at hand, I'd just pour olive oil, vinegar, salt, and pepper into the bowl of salad, then toss. Dinner was another large salad and steak or sautéed chicken and a glass of wine. I ate my daily ounce of nuts whenever I felt like it, and I often had a couple ounces of mozzarella string cheese. If I took my lunch to work, it could be as simple as a can of tuna (eaten with some tartar sauce), an ounce of nuts, and a couple ounces of cheese. Pretty simple if you ask me.

VINAIGRETTES

A homemade vinaigrette is an easy way to get your 2–3 tbsp (30–45 ml) of olive oil daily. The basic recipe is three parts olive oil to one part vinegar. Add salt, pepper, and other spices at your whim. Blend with a whisk, or put all ingredients in a jar with a lid and shake it. Favor red wine or white wine vinegar over balsamic. Balsamic has the highest carb content of the vinegars. I suppose you could use apple cider vinegar, too. See the Special Recipes section of this chapter for a couple fancy vinaigrettes. Mix a batch and keep it in the refrigerator— it should be good for a week. You may be able to find a commercially prepared vinaigrette in the salad dressing section of the supermarket. If so, be sure the oil is predominantly olive oil (not very common) and that a serving (usually 2 tbsp) has no more than 2 g of carb. Vinaigrettes can be used on salads, drizzled on cooked or fresh vegetables, and as marinades for fish, chicken, or beef.

If you're willing to do only minimal cooking, learn how to fry and scramble eggs. For extra credit, learn how to fry or grill steak or chicken, and sauté chicken and vegetables in olive oil.

TIME-SAVING CONVENIENCE

Canned meats and fish are times-savers and often less expensive than fresh, raw products. (Worried about mercury poisoning from fish? I've been practicing medicine for over two decades and haven't seen a case of it yet.) Canned sardines are available with sauces such as tomato, jalapeno, or mustard— just be sure it doesn't add more than a couple carb grams per 4-ounce (113 g) serving. Also watch out for added carbs in canned meats—chicken, for example. Man-made processed meats—sausages, Spam, bacon, or ham, for example—may have unacceptably high added carbs: if it's got over 2–3 g of carbs per 3 or 4-ounce (85–113 g) serving, take a pass and stick with natural meats.

Canned vegetables are usually OK, too. Consider canned green beans, asparagus, and spinach, for example. These are often criticized for their salt content, but the Ketogenic and Low-Carb Mediterranean Diets are naturally low in salt and tend to lower blood pressure, so you don't have to worry about the salt in canned vegetables. Frozen vegetables are also conveniently boiled-in-the-bag or microwaved. (Oh, no . . . that's not cooking, is it?)

Finally, in 2011, the food manufacturers are responding to consumer requests for truly "natural" foods with less man-made ingredients such as high fructose corn syrup (HFCS; pure carbohydrate). Search the shelves of your supermarket and you'll find ketchup and picante sauce without HFCS.

A WEEK OF MENUS

Here are some meal ideas to get you started. Each day's menu conforms fairly well to the Ketogenic Mediterranean Diet. Digestible carb totals for each day are in the 20 to 30 gram range. Average daily calorie count is 1,850, with a range of 1,550 to 1,950. This is more than some will want or need— just eat until you're full, not stuffed, and save the leftovers for another day. Of the total calories, average daily contribution from carbohydrate is 8%, from fat is 65%, from protein is 22%, and from alcohol is 5%. Calorie contributions from fat and protein vary quite a bit more day-to-day than do calories from carbohydrate.

Regarding olive oil, I tend to prefer extra virgin olive oil over the others. My salt choice is often potassium chloride rather than sodium chloride (table salt), which may help prevent muscle cramps sometimes seen at the start of very-low-carb eating.

"Dinner" is the evening meal, by the way.

Day 1

Breakfast: Eggs and Bratwurst

3 large eggs
1.5 tbsp (22 ml) olive oil

salt and pepper
1 (66g) pre-cooked bratwurst

Sauté eggs in the olive oil, salt and pepper to taste. Microwave a pre-cooked bratwurst. Digestible carb grams: 2.

Lunch: Tossed Tuna Salad and Almonds

3.5 oz (100 g) lettuce
1.5 oz (42 g) chopped onion
5.5 oz (150 g) chunked tomatoes
5-oz can (140 g) of solid white albacore tuna packed
    in water (drain and discard the fluid)
1.5 tbsp (22 ml) extra virgin olive oil
½ tbsp (7.5 ml) balsamic vinegar
salt and pepper
1 oz (28 g) almonds

In a 3-qt (3 liter) bowl, put lettuce, onion, chunked tomatoes, and tuna (3.25 oz or 90 g at this point). Add the olive oil, balsamic vinegar, and salt and pepper to taste. Mix well with a fork. Enjoy almonds separately, before, during, or after salad. Digestible carb grams: 12.

Dinner: Steak and Mushrooms

1.5 tbsp (21 g or 22 ml) butter
2 tsp (10 ml) olive oil
6 oz (170 g) steak
5 oz (140 g) sliced white mushrooms
2 tsp (10 ml) Worcestershire sauce or A.1. Steak
    Sauce
5 oz (150 ml) red wine
salt and pepper

Grill or sauté (with olive oil or butter) the steak. Melt 1.5 tbsp (22 ml) of butter in pan, add mushrooms and cook over medium heat about 3 minutes, stirring frequently. Season steak and mushrooms with salt and pepper to taste. Enjoy steak with your favorite steak sauce or Worcestershire sauce, but no more than 2 g of carbs in the sauce (e.g., 2 tsp (10 ml) of A.1. Sauce or Lea & Perrins Worcestershire sauce has 2 g of carb). Digestible carb grams: 10.

Day 2

Breakfast: Mexican Eggs and Avocado

3 large eggs (50 g each)
1 tbsp (14 g or 15 ml) butter
½ cup (240 ml) Pico de Gallo a la Rosa (See Special
    Recipes at end of this chapter)
1 California avocado (135 g), peeled, seeded, and
    sliced
salt and pepper

Sauté eggs in butter. Top with ½ cup Pico de Gallo a la Rosa (see Special Recipes). May substitute for Pico de Gallo: any serving of commercial picante sauce with no more than 3 g of digestible carb (digestible carb grams = total carb grams in serving minus fiber grams in serving). Salt and pepper to taste. Digestible carb grams: 7.

Lunch: Tuna Salad Over Lettuce, with Walnuts

1 large egg (50 g)
3 oz (85 g) romaine lettuce
5-oz can of white albacore tuna packed in water
    (drain and discard the fluid)

½ oz (14 g) onion, diced (about 2 tbsp)
8-inch stalk (40 g or 20-cm stalk) of celery, diced
2 tbsp (30 ml) Miracle Whip Dressing or regular
    mayonnaise
salt and pepper
dash of lemon (optional)
1 oz (28 g) walnuts

Hard-boil a large egg, then peel and dice. Drain liquid off a 5-ounce can of white albacore tuna (net 3.5 oz or 100 g of fish); empty tuna into bowl. To bowl, add diced egg, diced onion, diced celery, and Miracle Whip Dressing or regular mayonnaise. Mix all together, with salt and pepper and/or a dash of lemon to taste. Place on bed of romaine lettuce. Enjoy walnuts around mealtime. Digestible carb grams: 9.

Dinner: Baked Trout with Snow Peas (sugar snap peas)

7 tbsp (100 g) extra virgin olive oil
5 garlic cloves (15 g), diced
1.5 tbsp (6 g) raw parsley, chopped
1 tsp (5 ml) salt
1 tsp (5 ml) black pepper
¾ fl oz (22 g or ml) lemon juice
4 leaves (1.5 g) fresh basil, chopped
16 oz (450 g) fresh trout
6 oz (170 g) snow peas (sugar snap peas)
5 oz (150 ml) white wine

This recipe provides *two* large servings of fish and *two* servings of snow peas.

In a glass or plastic bowl, mix 5 tbsp (70 g) of the extra virgin olive oil, 3 of the diced garlic cloves (9 g), the chopped raw parsley, salt, black pepper, the lemon juice, and the chopped basil. This is your marinade.

Place fresh trout filets in a medium sized (8–9" or 20–23 cm diameter) glass baking dish, then cover with marinade. Let sit in refrigerator for 1–2 hours, turning occasionally. Preheat oven to 375°F (190°C). Pull fish dish out of refrigerator once you start the preheat process. Cover glass dish with aluminum foil, then bake in oven for 20–40 minutes. Cooking time depends on your oven and the thickness of the fish. Thin filets about 1/2" (1.25 cm) thick may be done in 20–25 minutes. Thicker fish (1" or 2.5 cm)) may take 30–45 minutes. This is a judgment call. When done, it should flake apart readily with a fork. This works well for trout, salmon, cod, tilapia, and perhaps others. Consider squeezing fresh lemon juice on cooked fish for extra zing.

Now the snow peas. Snap off and discard both tips of the snow pea pods. Sauté 2 diced garlic cloves (6 g) in olive oil over medium heat until soft, perhaps a couple minutes. To the pan add the snow peas. Salt and pepper to taste. Stir snow peas often, if not continuously, while cooking over medium heat, about 3 minutes. Enjoy 5 oz (150 ml) white wine with your meal. Digestible carb grams in wine and half the fish, half the snow peas: 11.

Day 3

Breakfast: Bacon and Eggs

3 large eggs (50 g each)
1.5 tbsp (22 ml) olive oil
6 slices pork bacon, cured (about 50 g cooked)

Fry the eggs in olive oil. Bake or fry the bacon. Digestible carb grams: 2.

Lunch: Chicken Salad Over Mixed Greens

1 large egg (50 g)
4 oz (110 g) cooked, diced chicken (canned or
    freshly sautéed in olive oil)
½ oz (14 g) raw onion, diced (about 2 tbsp)
8-inch stalk (40 g or 20-cm stalk) of raw celery,
    diced
2.5 tbsp (40 ml) Miracle Whip Dressing or regular
    Mayonnaise
2 oz (60 g) romaine lettuce
2 oz (60 g) raw baby spinach
1 oz (28 g) almonds
salt and pepper

Hard-boil an egg, then peel and dice. In a bowl, place the chicken and add the egg, onion, celery, and Miracle Whip Dressing or regular mayonnaise. Mix all together, with salt and pepper and/or a dash of lemon juice to taste. Place on bed of lettuce and baby spinach. Enjoy almonds around mealtime or later as a snack. Digestible carb grams: 10.

Dinner: Baked Balsamic Salmon and Green Beans

16 oz (450 g) salmon filets
salt and pepper
4 cloves (12 g) garlic, minced
1 tbsp (15 ml) olive oil
1.5 oz (45 ml) white wine for the glaze
4.5 tsp (22 ml) mustard
4 tbsp (60 ml) balsamic vinegar
1 tbsp (15 ml) granulated Splenda (or 1 packet (1g)
    of tabletop Splenda)
1.5 tbsp (22 ml) fresh chopped oregano (or 1 tsp
    (5 ml) dried oregano)
200 g canned green beans (or fresh green beans
    sautéed in olive oil/garlic)

5 oz (150 ml) dry white wine

This makes two large servings.

Preheat oven to 400°F (200°C). Line a baking sheet or pan (8" or 20 cm) with aluminum foil. Lightly salt and pepper the fish in the lined pan, with the skin side down.

Now the glaze. Sauté the minced garlic in olive oil in a small saucepan over medium heat for about three minutes, until it's soft. Then add and mix white wine (1.5 oz), mustard, vinegar, granulated Splenda, and 1/8 tsp (0.625 ml) salt. Simmer uncovered over low or medium heat until slightly thickened, about three minutes. Remove glaze from heat and spoon about half of it into a separate container for later use.

Drizzle and brush the salmon in the pan with the glaze left in the saucepan. Sprinkle the oregano on top.

Bake the fish in the oven for about 10–13 minutes, or until it flakes easily with a fork. Cooking time depends on your oven and thickness of the fish. Overcooking the fish will toughen it and dry it out. When done, use a turner to transfer the fish to plates, leaving the skin on the foil if able. Drizzle the glaze from the separate container over the filets with a spoon, or brush it on. Don't use the unwashed brush you used earlier on the raw fish.

Heat canned green beans (200 g) on stovetop or serve at room temperature straight out of the can.

Enjoy a 5-oz glass of dry white wine with your meal. This recipe makes two servings of fish and green beans. Digestible carb grams in wine, half the fish, half the green beans: 14.

[The *balsamic* vinegar adds six g of carb to each serving. To reduce vinegar carbs to zero, you could try this recipe with red wine vinegar, white wine vinegar, or cider vinegar. I've not tried that. Digestible carbs per serving would drop to 8 g.]

Day 4

Breakfast: Steak and Avocado

4 oz (110 g) raw steak
1 California avocado, peeled, seeded, and sliced
    (136 g)
½ tbsp (7 ml) olive oil (optional)
salt and pepper
1 tbsp (15 ml) vinaigrette (see Special Recipes) or
    commercial Italian dressing (regular, not low-fat,
    with less than 2 g of carb per tbsp or 15 ml)

Cook the steak over medium heat, adding half a tbsp (7 ml) olive oil at the start if desired. Salt and pepper to taste. Peel and slice a California avocado. Dress avocado with homemade vinaigrette (see Special Recipes) or commercial Italian dressing. Salt and pepper to taste. Digestible carb grams: 4.

Lunch: Aguacate Cucumber Salad

5 oz (140 g) cucumber, peeled and sliced into
    rounds
1 California avocado, peeled, seeded, and sliced
    (136 g)
2 tbsp (30 ml) AMD vinaigrette (see Special Recipes)
    or commercial Italian dressing described below

salt and pepper
dash of lime or lemon juice (optional)
1 oz walnuts

Mix the cucumber and avocado in a bowl with the AMD vinaigrette or commercial Italian dressing (regular, not low-fat, with 3 g or fewer carbs per 2 tbsp or 30 ml). Salt and pepper to taste. For extra zing, add a dash of lemon or lime juice. Enjoy the walnuts on the side now, or mid-afternoon as a snack. Digestible carb grams: 10.

Dinner: Bacon Shrimp Salad

2 slices (15 g) pork bacon, cured, cooked (or substitute 2 tbsp (30 ml) commercial real bacon bits)
2 tbsp (30 ml) AMD vinaigrette (see Special Recipes) or commercial Italian dressing as below
½ packet of tabletop Splenda
4 oz (110 g) fresh baby spinach
4 oz (110 g) cooked shrimp [Consider commercial pre-cooked, peeled shrimp to save time.]
6 oz (180 ml) dry white wine

Cook two bacon slices over medium heat, then crumble or cut in to tiny pieces (or substitute commercial real bacon bits). Add a half packet of Splenda to the AMD vinaigrette or commercial Italian dressing (regular, not low-fat, with 3 g or fewer carbs per 2 tbsp or 30 ml), then mix. On a bed of fresh baby spinach, place the cooked shrimp, then top with bacon pieces and vinaigrette. Enjoy with 6 oz dry white wine. Digestible carb grams: 9.

Day 5

Breakfast: Mexican Scrambled Eggs

4 large eggs (50 g each)
1.5 tbsp (22 ml) olive oil
4 tbsp (60 ml) Pico de Gallo a la Rose (see Special
    Recipes) or commercial picante sauce (having 2 g
    or fewer carbs per 2 tbsp)
salt and pepper

Whisk the eggs until smooth, add salt and pepper to taste; set aside. Heat the olive oil in a medium-sized frying pan then add the eggs and cook until done, scrambling now and then. Transfer to plate and top with 4 tbsp (60 ml) Pico de Gallo a al Rosa. Digestible carb grams: 6.

Lunch: Low-Carb Chili

1 cup (240 ml) Low-Carb Chili (see Special Recipes)
1 oz (28 g) almonds

Enjoy 1 oz of almonds around mealtime or later as a snack. Digestible carb grams: 13.

Dinner: Shark and Broccoli

4 oz (110 g) shark, raw
2 cloves (3 g) garlic, peeled and diced
3 tbsp (45 ml) olive oil
1.5 cups (150 g) chopped raw broccoli
salt and pepper
6 oz (180 ml) dry white wine

Lightly salt and pepper the shark, then set aside. Sauté the garlic in 2 tbsp (30 cc) of the olive oil a few minutes over medium heat. Then add the broccoli and sauté to your preference, adding salt and pepper to taste. Remove to a dish. Add another 1 tbsp (15 ml) olive oil to the pan and sauté the shark at medium heat until done, careful not to overcook. Enjoy with dry white wine. Digestible carb grams: 11.

Day 6

Breakfast: Chicken Salad Over Greens

1 large egg (50 g)
5-oz can (150 g) of cooked chicken (drain and
    discard liquid)
½ oz (14 g) onion (2 tbsp or 30 ml), diced
½ stick (40 g) of celery, diced
2 tbsp (30 ml) Miracle Whip Salad Dressing or
    Regular mayonnaise (not low-fat)
salt and pepper
2 oz (60 g) romaine lettuce
2 oz (60 g) raw baby spinach
dash of lemon or lime juice (optional)
1 oz (28 g) walnuts

Hard-boil the large egg, then peel and dice. Place the chicken into a bowl then add the egg, diced onion, diced celery, and the Miracle Whip Salad Dressing. Mix all together, with salt and pepper and/or a dash of lemon or lime juice to taste. Place on bed of romaine lettuce and fresh baby spinach. Enjoy walnuts around mealtime or later as a snack. Digestible carb grams: 11.

Lunch: Kippered Herring and Cheese

3.5 oz (100 g) canned herring
3 oz (80 g) cheese

Digestible carb grams: 2.

Dinner: Hamburger and Salad

8 oz (225 g) raw hamburger meat
1 oz (28 g) onion, finely chopped
1 tbsp (15 ml) A.1. Steak Sauce or Worcestershire
   sauce
salt and pepper
3 oz (85 g) lettuce
3 oz (85 g) tomato, cut into chunks
2 oz (60 g) cucumber, peeled and sliced
1.5 tbsp (22 ml) olive oil
½ tbsp (7 ml) vinegar

To the raw hamburger meat, add the chopped onion, A.1. Steak Sauce or Worcestershire sauce, and salt and pepper to taste. Blend thoroughly with your hands. (No particular need for *lean* hamburger; it's your choice.) Cook in pan over medium heat. While cooking, prepare your salad.

In a bowl, place the lettuce, tomato chunks, sliced cucumber, and finally, the olive oil and vinegar. Mix salad thoroughly. Salt and pepper to taste.

Enjoy with 6 oz of red wine. Digestible carb grams: 13.

Day 7

Breakfast: Brats and Tomatoes

6 oz (170 g) tomato, sliced

2 tbsp (30 ml) AMD vinaigrette (see Special Recipes) or commercial Italian dressing (regular, not low-fat, with 3 g or fewer carbs per 2 tbsp or 30 ml)

salt and pepper

2 pre-cooked bratwursts (about 2.3 oz or 65 g each)

6 tsp (30 ml) mustard (optional)

Dress the tomato slices with the vinaigrette, plus salt and pepper to taste. Heat 2 pre-cooked bratwursts as instructed on package. Use mustard on the brats if desired. Digestible carb grams: 8.

Lunch: Easy Tuna Plus Pecans

5-oz can (140 g) of albacore tuna

2 tbsp (30 ml) Miracle Whip Salad Dressing (or real, high-fat mayonnaise)

1 tsp (5 ml) lemon or lime juice

1 oz (28 g) pecan halves

Drain the liquid off the can of tuna then place tuna in a bowl. Add Miracle Whip Salad Dressing and lemon or lime juice. Mix thoroughly and enjoy. Eat 1 oz of pecan halves around mealtime or later as a snack. If you want to simplify this, forget the Miracle Whip and lemon; just use 1 oz (28 g) of commercial tartar sauce that derives at least 80% of calories from fat and has less than 3 g of carb per 2 tbsp or 30 ml. Digestible carb grams: 5.

Dinner: Ham Salad

2 oz (60 g) cooked ham, cut in to small cubes

1 oz (28 g) celery, sliced and diced

1 oz (28 g) seedless grapes (about 4 grapes), cut into
small chunks
1 oz (28 g) walnuts, coarsely crumbled
4 oz (110 g) romaine lettuce
3 tbsp AMD vinaigrette or commercial Italian,
   French, or ranch dressing having 2 or fewer
   grams of carb per 2 tbsp or 30 ml)

Lay out a bed of lettuce then sprinkle these on top:
ham, celery, grapes, walnuts. Finish construction
with AMD vinaigrette or commercial dressing. You're
done. Alternatively, substitute cooked chicken or
steak for ham. With chicken, apple may work better
than grapes. If having a glass of wine (6 fl oz or 180
ml) with meal, delete the grapes or the carb count
will be too high. Digestible carb grams: 10.

(When commercial dressing is used, the digestible
carb count is closer to 13 than 10 g.)

SPECIAL RECIPES

Nutrient analysis of these recipes is compliments of
SELF-NutritionData. You can analyze your own rec-
ipes there, finding the amounts of 40+ nutrients.
The web address is http://nutritiondata.self.com/.

ARIZONA'S BAKED CHEESECAKE

My daughter, Arizona, enjoys baking. I'm nudging
her into low-carb baking since I miss my sweets.

Arizona usually prepares the commercial cheese-
cakes based on a pre-mixed box: you add some
fresh ingredients, mix, then refrigerate. The baked
cheesecake here is more work, but I think well
worth the effort. We had fun making this together.

Ingredients for crust:

1.5 cups (226 g) ground nuts (pecan, walnut, or almond)
5.5 tbsp (82 ml) melted butter
½ tsp (2 g) ground cinnamon
1 egg white (33 g)
1 tbsp (15 ml) Granulated Splenda No Calorie Sweetener (optional)

Ingredients for filling:

24 oz (675 g) cream cheese
1 cup (230 g) sour cream
4 large eggs (50 g each)
1 cup (28 g) Granulated Splenda No Calorie Sweetener
juice from one lemon (47 g or ml)
2 tsp (10 ml) vanilla extract

Preparation

Have the following ingredients at room temperature before you start: eggs, cream cheese, sour cream.

Preheat oven to 350°F (175°C).

First, the crust. Put ground pecans, 4 tbsp (60 ml) of the melted butter (fine to microwave briefly), cinnamon, granulated Splenda, and egg white in bowl, then blend all. Spread onto bottom of greased (with melted butter, the last 1.5 tbsp or 22 ml) 9" (20–25 cm) springform pan. Cover with plastic wrap to aid spreading evenly; remove and discard plastic wrap after spreading the crust. Bake in 350°F (175°C) oven for 10–15 minutes then remove. Then reduce heat to 325°F (160°C).

Filling: Use a mixer on low to medium setting to beat the cream cheese until fluffy. Blend in the Splenda incrementally, a little at a time, beating until creamy. Then mix in the lemon juice and vanilla extract. Gently mix in one egg at a time and beat on low speed after each egg. Mix in the sour cream last. Pour cream cheese mixture into the crusted spring-form pan. Place on the top rack in the 325°F (160°C) preheated oven for 50–60 minutes. On the rack below that, place a pie pan full of water. [The water pan and gentle handling of the eggs help prevent cracking of the final product.] When time is up, turn off the oven and open the oven door but leave the cake in the oven to cool slowly. After an hour, remove from oven. After it cools to room temperature, put it in the refrigerator to age for 24 hours.

Notes:

■ The filling has one cup of Splenda, which I estimate is one ounce (28 g). This has 96 calories, which I assume is mostly from maltodextrin rather than sucralose.

■ Many cooks just use a glass pie pan instead of the springform pan. The volume of this recipe is likely too much for a 9" (23 cm) pie pan, so you could reduce the amounts; or make a larger pie or two smaller ones.

■ Some cooks don't bother to bake the crust first.

■ Reduce the carb count even further by omitting the crust.

■ For higher fiber, substitute flax meal for about a third or ½ of the ground nuts.

■ The Splenda in this recipe is not the same as in the individual serving packets.

Nutrient analysis:

Recipe makes 12 servings. Each serving has 444 calories, 8 g carbohydrate, 2 g fiber, 6 g digestible carbohydrate, 8 g protein, 43 g fat. 6% of calories are from carbohydrate, 8% from protein, 86% from fat.

LOW-CARB CHILI

It's spicy, but not hot spicy. Peeled and sliced cold cucumbers make a nice side dish. If your children or housemates aren't eating low-carb, they may enjoy the chili mixed 50:50 with cheese macaroni, and buttered cornbread on the side.

Ingredients

20 oz (567 g) raw ground beef, 80% lean meat/20% fat
20 oz (567 g) raw pork Italian sausage
1 large onion
14.5 oz (411 g) canned diced tomatoes
4 oz (113 g) tomato paste
1 tbsp (15 ml) dry unsweetened cocoa powder
5 garlic cloves
½ tsp (2.5 ml) salt
¼ tsp (1.2 ml) ground allspice
2 tbsp (30 ml) chili powder
¼ tsp (1.2 ml) ground cinnamon
½ tbsp (7.5 ml) ground cumin
¼ tsp (1.2 ml) ground cayenne pepper
2 packets (1 g per packet) Splenda tabletop sweetener
1 cup (240 ml) water

Preparation

Cut the Italian sausage into small pieces. Sauté the sausage, ground beef, onions, and garlic in a large pot. Don't just brown the meat, cook it thoroughly. When done, drain off the fat if desired. Add the remainder of ingredients, bring to a boil, then simmer for about an hour. Add additional water if the chili looks too thick. Makes eight cups. Serving size is one cup (240 ml).

Nutrient Analysis:

Recipe makes 8 servings of 1 cup (240 ml). Each serving has 492 calories, 14 g carbohydrate, 3 g fiber, 11 g digestible carbohydrate, 24 g protein, 38 g fat. 10% of calories are from carbohydrate, 21% from protein, 69% from fat.

Notes: Analysis is based on fat not being drained from the cooked meat. Calorie count and calories from fat would be a bit lower if you drained off fat.

PICO DE GALLO A LA ROSA

Try this, for example, over fried eggs.

Ingredients

6 oz (170 g) tomatoes
2 oz (56 g) onion
1 jalapeno pepper (14 g)
3–4 tbsp (2 g) cilantro
salt

Preparation

Chop all vegetables very finely. Use the entire jala-peno, including seeds, but not the stem. If you pre-fer less spicy heat, use less jalapeno and discard the seeds. Combine all ingredients after chopping. Salt to taste. Eat at room temperature, chilled, or heated at medium heat in a saucepan (about 5 minutes, until jalapenos lose their intense green color). Makes 1.25 cups.

Nutrient Analysis:

Recipe makes about three servings of ½ cup (120 ml) each. One serving has 80 calories, 4 g carb, 1 g fiber, 3 g digestible carb, 1 g protein, minimal fat. 83% of calories are from carbohydrate, 10% from protein, 7% from fat.

ALMOND POUND CAKE

My son, Paul, and I had a great time making this when he was 11-years-old, around the time he an-nounced he "might be interested in a career as a culinary professional." This cake was our first joint baking project.

2 cups (224 g) almond flour
½ cup (113 g) butter at room temperature
4 oz (116 g) cream cheese at room temperature
1 cup (28 g) Splenda Granulated No Calorie Swee-
    tener
6 eggs, medium size (44 g each), at room tempera-
    ture
1 tsp (5 ml) baking powder
1 tbsp (15 ml) lemon zest (or 1.5 tsp or 7 ml lemon
    extract)
1 tsp (5 ml) vanilla extract

If you can't find almond flour, make your own by grinding almonds into the consistency of a flour. You can do this in a blender or electric coffee bean grinder.

Preparation

Preheat oven to 350°F (175°C).

Mix the butter, cream cheese, and Splenda with a hand-held or table-top mixer, then beat in the eggs one at a time, mixing thoroughly after each egg. In a separate container, mix the baking powder into the almond flour. Add the almond flour a little at a time into the butter/sour cream bowl, beating as you go. Then mix in vanilla extract and lemon zest. Pour into a 9-inch (22-24 cm) cake pan greased with butter, vegetable oil, or Baker's Joy Baking Spray, then bake at 350°F (175°C). for 35-40 minutes.

Nutrient Analysis:

Recipe makes 12 servings. Each serving has 248 calories, 5 g carbohydrate, 1 g fiber, 4 g digestible carbohydrate, 5 g protein, 18 g fat. 27% of calories are from carbohydrate, 9% from protein, 64% from fat.

AMD VINAIGRETTE

Try this on salads, fresh vegetables, or as a marinade for chicken, fish, or beef. If using as a marinade, keep the entree/marinade combo in the refrigerator for 4–24 hours. Seasoned vinaigrettes taste even better if you let them sit for several hours after preparation. This recipe was in my first book, *The*

Advanced Mediterranean Diet; hence, "AMD vinaigrette."

Ingredients

1 clove (3 g) garlic
juice from ½ lemon (23 g or ml)
a third of a cup (78 ml) oil olive
2 tbsp (8 g) fresh parsley
½ tsp (2.5 ml)) salt
½ tsp (2.5 ml) yellow mustard
½ tsp (1.2 ml) paprika
2 tbsp (30 ml) vinegar, red wine,

Preparation

In a bowl, combine all ingredients and whisk together. Alternatively, you can put all ingredients in a jar with a lid and shake vigorously. Let sit at room temperature for an hour, for flavors to meld. Then refrigerate. It should "keep" for at least 5 days in refrigerator. Shake before using. Servings per batch: 3.

Nutrient Analysis:

Recipe makes 3 servings (2 tbsp or 30 ml per serving). Each serving has 220 calories, 2 g digestible carb, almost no fiber, negligible protein, 24 g fat. 3% of calories are from carbohydrate, 97% from fat.

MUSTARD VINAIGRETTE

Try this on salads, fresh vegetables, or as a marinade for chicken, fish, or beef. If using as a marinade, keep the entree/marinade combo in the refrigerator for 4–24 hours.

Ingredients

3 tsp (15 ml) yellow mustard, yellow
¾ cup (177 ml) olive oil
½ tsp (2.5 ml) salt
½ tsp (2.5 ml) pepper (fresh ground if available)
¼ cup (60 ml) cider vinegar

Preparation

Mix all ingredients in a jar with a lid. Shake vigorously to create an emulsion. Let sit at room temperature for an hour, for flavors to meld. Then refrigerate. Should "keep" for at least 5 days in refrigerator. Shake before using. Makes one cup.

Nutrient Analysis:

Recipe makes one cup (8 servings of 2 tbsp each). Each serving has 182 calories, negligible carbs, zero protein, 20 g fat. 1% of calories are from carbohydrate, 99% from fat.

You'll find sources of free online low-carb recipes in the next chapter.

8

Daily Life With Low-Carb Eating

I haven't scared you off yet, huh?

Great!

The program I've laid out presents some definite challenges, a few of which are unique. Think of them as opportunities for personal growth. But you don't have to go it alone, nor blaze any trails through uncharted territory. I'm here to help, as is a scattered online low-carb community.

This chapter will give you an approach to overcoming the common problems linked to low-carb eating. The coping mechanisms here are not exhaustive, and you will need, at times, to figure out for yourself what works for you and your unique metabolism.

In order, here's what's ahead:

1. Find more low-carb recipes
2. Short-term physical effects
3. Shopping for food
4. Dining out
5. Cheating
6. Sweet cravings
7. Holidays
8. Hunger
9. Record-keeping
10. Weight-loss tips
11. Miscellanea
12. Social issues

1. FIND MORE LOW-CARB RECIPES

Chapter seven has a few low-carb recipes, both in the "A Week of Meals" and "Special Recipes" sections. Find many more at free low-carb websites and online forums, such as:

- The message boards at Low Carb Friends (http://www.lowcarbfriends.com)
- Active Low-Carbers Forum (http://forum.lowcarber.org)
- Laura Dolson's About.com: Low Carb Diets blog (http://lowcarbdiets.about.com)
- Chef Barrae has posted hundreds of low-carb recipes (including nutritional analysis) at her blog: Unrestricted Tastes on Restricted Diets: Distinctive Diabetic Recipes (http://chefbarrae.blogspot.com).
- Jennifer Eloff has authored numerous low-carb cookbooks, starting with her flagship, *Splendid Low-Carbing*, followed by four others in the same vein. Jennifer generously

shares many of her fantastic recipes at her blog, Splendid Low-Carbing. Most of her recipes include some nutrient analysis, such as carb and calorie counts. Jennifer has a particular interest in cooking with Splenda, helping you satisfy your sweet tooth. Find her blog at (http://low-carb-news.blogspot.com/).

- DAR, a type 2 diabetic, offers her favorite low-carb recipes at http://dardreams.wordpress.com/. Nutrient analysis is limited to digestible carb grams, referred to as "net carbs."

- Dana Carpender has a number of great low-carb recipe books, such as the classic *500 Low-Carb Recipes*, as well as *200 Low-Carb Slow Cooker Recipes*, *15-Minute Low-Carb Recipes*, and *1001 Low-Carb Recipes*. Check out some of her free online recipes and purchase books at her blog, Hold the Toast! (http://holdthetoast.com/).

You need to know the digestible or net *carb grams* per serving of any recipe you try. If not provided for you, you can do a full nutritional analysis of any recipe at SELF-NutritionData (http://nutritiondata.self.com/).

2. SHORT-TERM PHYSICAL EFFECTS

Very-low-carb eating is quite safe in the vast majority of generally healthy people. However, you need to be aware of minor problems that may crop up.

121

INDUCTION FLU

This refers to a sense of mild malaise, easy-fatigue, low energy, achiness, and dizziness that often affects people switching from a carbohydrate-based energy metabolism to fat-based. Some folks have the entire syndrome, others just parts. It starts on the second or third day of the diet and may last for several days, a week at the most. People with diabetes need to make sure the symptoms are not caused by low blood sugar by using their home glucose monitor.

Regarding low energy and easy fatigue, people who are used to exercising or working vigorously may notice that they can't perform at their prior workload, an effect that may be noticeable for two to four weeks. They may need to cut back the intensity of their work-outs temporarily. The first few weeks of very-low-carb eating are not a good time to start a vigorous exercise program.

Induction flu is temporary. It's proof that your body is going through a watershed moment. Try to tough it out—you'll be glad you did.

LEG CRAMPS

These occur commonly in the first few weeks or months. They tend to happen at night, even waking people from sleep. While not serious, they can be painful. Cramps are often prevented by taking additional supplemental magnesium, potassium, calcium, or a combination. If they persist, see your doctor for a blood test of these minerals.

A stretching exercise may prevent leg cramps: 1) Stand about two or three feet away from a wall (measured at the toes) and keep your feet planted in one spot, 2) lean forward against the wall and use your outstretched arms and hands to keep your body from hitting the wall, 3) keeping your trunk and legs in a straight line, bend your elbows to let your head approach the wall, 4) notice the slight tensing and stretching of the calf muscles (this may be slightly uncomfortable but shouldn't be painful), 5) hold that position for 10 seconds, 6) then stand up straight and relax a while, 7) repeat steps 1 through 5 for five or ten times. For nocturnal leg cramps, do this stretching just before bedtime.

CONSTIPATION OR DIARRHEA

If a bowel problem occurs, it's more likely to be constipation related to lower-than-usual fiber consumption. Others have the opposite problem, diarrhea. You might be able to identify a specific food causing symptoms, such as cheese and constipation. Eliminate or cut back on the offending item. Sugar-free Metamucil powder—one teaspoon in water—once or twice daily usually resolves constipation. Or you could concentrate on the higher fiber vegetables.

LOW BLOOD SUGAR

Since ingested carbohydrates are normally the main source of blood sugar, cutting back drastically tends to reduce blood sugar levels, even in people who don't have diabetes or prediabetes. Symptoms of low blood sugar (hypoglycemia) are rare in healthy people starting a ketogenic diet. But hypoglycemia is much more common and potentially serious in diabetics taking certain medications. See chapter four for a thorough review.

LOW BLOOD PRESSURE

The Ketogenic Mediterranean Diet is relatively low in salt, which may explain why low blood pressure can occur. If you take drugs to lower your blood pressure, the dosage my need to be reduced to prevent excessively low blood pressure. Symptoms of low blood pressure include dizziness, lightheadedness, weakness, fainting, and fatigue. Note the similarity to induction flu. You may notice these only when going from sitting to standing, or from lying to standing.

If low blood pressure is causing the symptom, we usually find a systolic blood pressure under 90 mmHg. "Systolic pressure" is the top or first number in a blood pressure reading such as 125/85 (systolic pressure is 125). The only way to tell if the aforementioned symptoms are related to blood pressure is to check a blood pressure with an accurate monitor, which most of us don't have at home or work. Perhaps you could borrow a friend's. Alternatively, check your blood pressure at your doctor's office or one of the free machines in many pharmacies and supermarkets. In those settings, a systolic pressure under 100 mmHg, even if you feel fine, suggests that your pressure at other times is under 90. Low blood pressures often responds to an increase in salt and water consumption, such as half a teaspoon daily mixed in water or used on food.

3. SHOPPING

Finding food for the Ketogenic or Low-Carb Mediterranean Diet shouldn't be a problem. Specific recommended foods are readily available at supermarkets. People committed long-term to the low-carb way of eating often get into baking or cooking with low-carb components that may be a bit harder to find. An example is almond flour, used as a substitute for wheat flour in baking cookies and pastries, among other things. You may find low-carb products at local stores or available on the Internet (e.g., Netrition.com).

You'll find a grocery shopping list for the Ketogenic and Low-Carb Mediterranean Diets at this URL: http://advancedmediterraneandiet.com/printabledocuments.html.

How to choose a fresh fish for cooking:

1. Sniff it. Pass if it smells fishy, nasty, or pungent.
2. Check for clear, dark eyes. Pass if eyes are dull gray and sunken.
3. Does it look or feel slimy? Take a pass.
4. Skin should be moist and shiny, almost metallic.
5. Flesh should be firm, not mushy. Press it with your finger—it shouldn't leave an imprint.
6. Look for bright red gills.
7. Cook within a day or two.

Keep your refrigerator and cupboards stocked with the foods you'll be eating, particularly if others in your household are eating regular high-carb foods that will tempt you.

4. DINING OUT

You'll be tempted to return to "normal" high-carb eating especially when you're away from your home's well-stocked cupboards and refrigerator. Be ready to deal with it.

One option is to take your food with you. For road trips, take nuts, dark chocolate, canned fish and meat, vegetables, an ice cooler stocked with cheese, condiments, vegetables, and your favorite no- or low-carb drinks. (My family likes to stay at motels with "free breakfast," but that too often means the only low-carb offerings are butter and half-n-half coffee creamer.)

Buffets will have several low-carb options for you.

Fast-food restaurants also offer several low-carb options. Order a burger and throw away the bun—or they may build the burger for you wrapped in lettuce. Eat the topping of pizza, not the bread. Fancy salads topped with chicken or beef are commonly available. Nearly all fast-food restaurants provide nutritional analysis for menu items—ask for it if you aren't sure of the carb count.

5. CHEATING

Let's face it: everybody cheats on diets.

It's easier to deal with the truth when you recognize the truth. It's not going to be the end of the world if you go "off plan" for one or two days a year and just eat like everyone else around you. I'm not suggesting pigging out as if you were at a decadent ancient Roman feast. Just eat reasonable amounts of regular, carb-rich foods. You'll probably gain a pound or two (up to a kilogram). Returning to a strict Ketogenic Mediterranean Diet and exercising a little more for a few days will usually resolve the extra weight.

A more common issue is that someone has a craving for a particular food and can't live with the possibility of never eating it again. For instance, I love apple pie and Cinnabon cinnamon rolls; I'd get depressed if I could never again have them. So what I'll do, perhaps every couple months, is have the cinnamon roll (730 calories!) or a large serving of apple pie *instead of a meal*. Call it a "cheat meal." I eat low-carb, maybe even lower than usual, for the remainder of that day. What about eating your usual three daily meals *plus* the cinnamon roll, and just burn off the extra calories with exercise? Sounds logical. But a 150-pound person (68 kg) would need to jump rope for four and a half hours to burn 730 calories. I won't do that, and you won't either.

Cheat days and cheat meals don't work for everyone. Think about alcoholics who have stopped drinking. Standard advice from addiction specialists—and I agree—is that alcoholics should *never* again drink alcohol. Not even a sip. Probably not even non-alcoholic "beer." That's because it's too tempting and could trigger a drinking binge that could be life-threatening. A few people are that way with carbohydrates. You could say they're addicted. They shouldn't have cheat days or cheat meals. Does this apply to you? Only you can answer that.

Of course, a meal or entire day with more than the usual amount of carb consumption can play havoc with blood sugar levels, which is a major potential problem in diabetes. It's generally more of a problem in type 1 diabetes than type 2. (Prediabetics will have higher blood sugars, but rarely know it or suffer acute consequences.) If you have diabetes and plan on cheating now and then, plan ahead. Ask your doctor or diabetes nurse educator how you could handle temporarily higher blood sugars. Don't worry about being judged harshly; experienced clinicians know that diet compliance is never perfect. [I'm convinced a fair number of my diabetic patients pretty much eat what they want most of the time!]

Management options include: 1) taking more insulin or other diabetic drugs, 2) adding some exercise—perhaps intense and prolonged—after the high-carb meal, 3) skipping the next meal, 4) eating the extra carbs before mid-afternoon so that physical activity later in the day will "burn up" the extra blood sugar, or 5) just living with temporarily high blood sugars.

Some diabetics decide it's just not worth the worry and hassle to plan for a cheat day or cheat meal. They just stay "on plan." More power to you! They often opt for low-carb versions of regular foods (see section 1 earlier in this chapter for recipes).

6. SWEET CRAVINGS

If sweets are your downfall, be aware that cravings tend to dissipate after several months of low-carbing. It may take up to a year. Unfortunately, that doesn't happen for everyone.

If your cravings persist and you can't resist them, your best option is artificial sweeteners, sometimes known as sugar substitutes. Examples are sucralose, aspartame, sorbitol, erythritol, and stevia. Several of these can be used in cooking and baking.

Online low-carb recipe repositories will have many sweet options. Or use off-the-shelf prepared items from grocery stores. Try sugar-free gelatin or sugar-free hard candy.

I have no objection if you wish to drink one or two diet soda pops a day. Water may be better for you.

7. HOLIDAYS

Holidays like Thanksgiving (in the U.S.) and Christmas present major temptations to folks trying to limit carb consumption. It's easier to stay "on plan" if you don't socialize much, but most of us visit relatives or others, and the temptation to eat like everyone else is great and often irresistible.

Sometimes people almost "force" carbs on you. For diabetics and prediabetics, you can often say, "No, thanks. My doctor has me on a special diet," and that should be the end of it. Others don't wish to reveal a medical condition and can say, "I'm fine, thank you. I just feel better if I eat a different way," or, "I'm fine, thank you. I'm not hungry right now." Still others are just totally honest and open and say, "No, thanks. That makes my blood sugar spike way too high."

Another option is to cheat on the diet.

8. HUNGER

If you get hungry between meals, choose an item from the "unlimited" foods list and see if that helps. Or eat cheese, up to three ounces a day. A can of tuna or a couple hard-boiled eggs may not be your traditional snacks, but they aren't likely to blow your blood sugar control or weight management plan compared to a bag of corn chips or handful of cookies

9. RECORD-KEEPING

You can track your weight, blood sugars, and consumption of the major food items with the "KMD & LCMD Daily Log" available for free at http://advancedmediterraneandiet.com/printabledocuments.html.

If desired, you can pretty easily keep track of your daily consumption online at SELF-NutritionData. The web address is http://nutritiondata.self.com/. First, register your free membership. Then go to the "My ND" section near the top of the page and click on "My Recipes." Make each of your days a single recipe with a title such as "LCMD Day 1." Enter everything you eat in the course of a day. Remember to click "Save" before you leave that day's recipe. At the end of the day, choose the "Save and Analyze" button. You'll get a comprehensive nutritional analysis of that day's consumption.

And I mean *comprehensive*: overall percentages of carbohydrate, protein, and fat, along with total calories and 40 or 50 vitamins, minerals, and other nutrients.

If you're going to do this for more than a couple days, use the "My Foods" feature and you'll end up saving time. An exercise like this—essentially a food diary—over four or five days is also helpful in figuring out why weight loss may have stalled or blood sugars are getting higher. Carb consumption often creeps up unnoticed, and at a certain point will sabotage the best-laid plans.

You can do similar record-keeping and nutritional analysis at FitDay (http://fitday.com/). FitDay also helps you easily track your weight and exercise and estimate calories burned exercising. It's definitely worth a look. It's free.

Yet another good option for record-keeping is Calorie Count (http://caloriecount.about.com/). It's free, too.

Both Calorie Count and FitDay have active community forums for support and education. They are not designed specifically for diabetics, however.

10. WEIGHT-LOSS TIPS

Record-keeping is often the key to success. For options, see the section immediately preceding this.

Accountability is another key to success. Consider documenting your program and progress on a free website such as FitDay, SparkPeople, 3FatChicks, or others. If your initiation to low-carb eating is a major undertaking (and it should be) consider blogging about your adventure on a free platform such as Wordpress or Blogger. Such a public commitment may be just what you need to keep you motivated.

Do you have a friend or spouse who wants to lose weight? Start the same program at the same time and support each other. That's built-in accountability.

If you tend to over-eat, floss and brush your teeth after you're full. You'll be less likely to go back for more anytime soon.

Eat at least two or three meals daily. Skipping meals may lead to uncontrollable overeating later on. On the other hand, ignore the diet gurus who say you *must* eat every two or three hours.

Eat meals at a leisurely pace, chewing and enjoying each bite thoroughly before swallowing.

Plan to give yourself a specific reward for every 10 pounds (4.5 kg) of weight lost. You know what you like. Consider a weekend get-away, a trip to the beauty salon, jewelry, an evening at the theater, a professional massage, home entertainment equipment, new clothes, etc.

Carefully consider when would be a good time to start your new lifestyle. It should be a period of low or usual stress. Bad times would be Thanksgiving day, Christmas/New Years' holiday, the first day of a Caribbean cruise, and during a divorce.

If you know you've eaten enough at a meal to satisfy your nutritional requirements yet you still feel hungry, drink a large glass of water and wait a while.

Limit television to less than a few hours a day.

Maintain a consistent eating pattern throughout the week and year.

Eat breakfast routinely.

Control emotional eating.

Weigh frequently: daily during active weight-loss efforts and during the first two months of your maintenance-of-weight-loss phase. After that, cut back to weekly weights if you want. Daily weights will remind you how hard you worked to achieve your goal.

Be aware that you might regain five or 10 pounds of fat now and then. You probably will. Don't freak out. It's human nature. You're not a failure; you're human. But draw the line and get back on the old Ketogenic Mediterranean Diet for one or two months. Analyze and learn from the episode. Why did it happen? Slipping back into your old ways? Slacking off on exercise? Too many special occasion feasts or cheat days? Allowing junk food or non-essential carbs back into the house?

Learn which food item is your nemesis—the food that consistently torpedoes your resolve to eat right. For example, mine is anything sweet. Remember an old ad campaign for a potato chip: "Betcha can't eat just one!"? Well, I can't eat just one cookie. So I don't get started. I might eat one if it's the last one available. Or I satisfy my sweet craving with a diet soda, piece of dark chocolate, or sugar-free gelatin. Just as a recovering alcoholic can't drink any alcohol, perhaps you should totally abstain from...? You know your own personal gastronomic Achilles heel. Or heels. Experiment with various strategies for vanquishing your nemesis.

11. Miscellanea

Use a food scale and measuring devices to improve your compliance with portion sizes, especially during the first month. Thereafter you may be able to judge portion size by eye and feel.

One ounce (28 g) of cheese is about the size of a domino.

An ounce (28 g) of nuts is about a quarter of a cup, or a heap of nuts in the palm of your hand, not covering your fingers.

Fish and poultry may be a little more healthful for you than red meat.

Regular meat products may be a little healthier than processed meats like bacon, bologna and other luncheon meats, pre-cooked commercial sausages, etc.

As long as a food is low-carb, don't go for the low-fat version. For instance, low-fat yogurt is over-loaded with carbohydrates compared to the full-fat version.

Tell your housemates you are on a special diet and ask for their support. You may also need to tell your co-workers and others with whom you spend significant time. If they care about you, they'll be careful not to tempt you off the diet.

Do your grocery shopping from a list.

For help with basic culinary skills, peruse these books: How *to Cook Everything: Simple Recipes for Great Food*, by Mark Bittman; *Joy of Cooking: 75th Anniversary Edition*, by Irma S. Rombauer, Marion Rombauer Becker, and Ethan Becker; *Betty Crocker Cookbook: Everything You Need to Know to Cook Today.*

12. SOCIAL ISSUES

AGAINST THE GRAIN OF A CARB-CENTRIC CULTURE

There was a time in my life that I just loved whole grain bread, pizza, and pasta. I couldn't imagine life without them. As an experiment, I went an entire year eating low-carb, without whole grain bread, pizza, and pasta. At that point, I didn't miss them much at all. I realized I could easily have a happy, healthy, fulfilling, life without whole grain bread, pizza, and pasta. If you told me I had a medical condition that would worsen if I ate them, I could easily live without them and not complain.

During that same experimental year, I cut way back on my consumption of sweet fruits, starchy vegetables, and sweets (cookies, cakes, candy bars, pies). After the year was up, I didn't miss the sweet fruits and starchy vegetables, although I did miss my sweet things. I could see living the rest of my life without sweet fruits and starchy vegetables. Giving up apple pie and Cinnabon cinnamon rolls would be tougher.

That's just my experience, but I'm not alone. I wouldn't ask you to give up many of your beloved carbohydrates if I didn't know it was possible, and that others had done it successfully. The trade-offs for many of us will be improved health and slimmer waistlines.

The odd thing about the Ketogenic and Low-Carb Mediterranean Diets is that they go against the grain (pun intended) of the Western food culture that prominently features carbohydrates. Anyone following the diet is immediately in a strange position, surrounded continuously with opportunities and inducements to consume carbs. Especially nutrient-depleted, highly refined carbs such as white bread, sugar, flour, fruit juice, potato and corn chips, high fructose corn syrup, and soda pop.

It's difficult to be immersed in such a culture, especially for a diabetic or prediabetic who may have lived happily and healthfully in that society for 40 years before diagnosis. Old habits are hard to break. Food preferences are deeply ingrained from an early age.

The only way I know to counteract that cultural pull is to take to heart the medical consequences of continued participation in that poisonous environment. Frankly, it's not going to matter much if your blood sugar *today* is 211 mg/dl versus 93 mg/dl (11.7 mmol/l versus 5.2 mmol/l). But if that difference is sustained over years, you're putting yourself at risk for all the usual diabetic complications that would degrade the quality and duration of your life.

How do you motivate someone today to make a radical change in behavior that may not have a pay-off for another decade or more? Education is the only tactic I know that works consistently. People are more receptive when they're hospitalized with diabetic symptoms and blood sugars are 450 mg/dl (25 mmol/l). Even then change it's often a struggle.

Millions of people with normal carbohydrate metabolism have used very-low-carb eating as a way to lose excess weight and keep it off. It's a little easier for diabetics and prediabetics to stick with it in light of the potential health and longevity benefits. Low-carbing for them is not so much a lifestyle choice as it is a medical necessity.

Low-carb eating increasingly will be seen as viable and healthful as news of recent scientific developments becomes mainstream (see Annotated Bibliography). Low-carbing will be easier to maintain then, diabetic or not.

The Low-Carb Mediterranean Diet is a radical departure from the way most people are used to eating. Too radical, perhaps, for a majority of diabetics and prediabetics to sustain for a lifetime. I can't guarantee a diabetic will live longer or have fewer complications by following it. I can guarantee it's what I'd do if I had diabetes or prediabetes myself. For most followers, it will result in blood sugar levels much closer to the normal range, compared to the way most people with diabetes eat in 2011.

But enough philosophizing.

ONLINE SUPPORT

If you feel lonely and odd eating very-low-carb, you will find copious online support at the Low Carb Friends message boards (http://lowcarbfriends.com/) and Active Low-Carbers Forum (http://forum.lowcarber.org/). There are plenty of low-carbers also on the forums at FitDay, Spark-People, and 3FatChicks.

PARTIES AND HOLIDAY MEALS

In general, I think it's a good idea to let those around you know that you're eating low-carb. I understand there may be good reasons to keep it a secret, however. If you're not in charge of the food, let the host know you'll be focusing on meat, chicken, eggs, fish, cheese, and low-carb vegetables. The meats are usually main courses anyway. You'll simply not be eating many of the side dishes like bread, potatoes, corn, peas, and desserts. If you're the host, I'm sure you'll want to provide your guests—especially children—with the usual high-carb fare. With some experience, you could serve adults a delicious low-carb feast without their awareness.

If the host is a vegetarian or vegan serving his usual cuisine, you may not be able to low-carb. Think about eating before the event, and then just eat a little to be cordial.

9

Prepare For Weight Loss

Did you know that four of every 10 women in the U.S. are trying to lose weight? The figure for men is one in three.

Among diabetics and prediabetics, at least eight of every 10 are carrying excess body fat. Losing the fat counteracts insulin resistance and makes it easier to control blood sugars with minimal diabetic medication.

Are you ready to lose the excess weight once and for all? It's crept up on you over the last few years, or longer. Permanent weight loss is not easy and can't be done on a whim. Success requires careful forethought.

Individuals lucky enough to be generally healthy and free of diabetes and prediabetes have more choices, which can be confusing. They must ask themselves, "which of the myriad weight-loss programs will I follow? Can I design my own program? Should I use a diet book? Sign up for Nutri-System, Weight Watchers, or Jenny Craig? Should I stop wasting my time dieting and go directly to bariatric surgery? Can I simply cut back on sodas and chips? What should I eat? What should I not eat? Do I need to start exercising? What kind? How much? Do I need to join a gym? What methods are proven to increase my odds of success? How much weight should I lose? Should I use weight-loss pills or supplements? Which ones? What's the easiest, most effective way to lose weight? Is there a program that doesn't require willpower? Now, what were those 'top 10 super-power foods' that melt away the fat? Am I ready to get serious and stick with it this time?"

For people with diabetes and prediabetes, losing weight with a very-low-carb ketogenic diet is one of the best ways to do it. It directly addresses the fundamental metabolic abnormality in these disorders: abnormal carbohydrate handling. The ketogenic diet kills two birds with one stone: excess weight and high blood sugars.

MOTIVATION

Immediate, short-term motivation to lose weight may stem from an upcoming high school reunion, swimsuit season, or a wedding. You want to look your best. Maybe you want to attract a mate or keep one interested. Perhaps a boyfriend, co-worker, or relative said something mean about your weight.

These motivators may work, but only temporarily. Basing a lifestyle change on them is like building on shifting sands. You need a firmer foundation for a lasting structure. Without a lifestyle change, you're unlikely to vanquish a chronic overweight problem. Proper long-term motivation may grow from:

- the discovery that you feel great and have more energy when you are lighter and eating sensibly
- the sense of accomplishment from steady progress
- the acknowledgment that you have free will and are responsible for your weight and many aspects of your health
- the inspiration from seeing others take charge of their lives successfully
- the admission that you have some guilt and shame about being fat, and that you like yourself more when you're not fat [I'm not laying shame or guilt on you; many of us do it to ourselves.]
- the awareness of overweight-related adverse health effects and their improvement with even modest weight loss

Appropriate motivation will support the commitment and willpower that will be needed for success.

I'm thinking of how Dave Ramsey, when he's counseling people who have gotten way overhead in debt, tells them they have to get mad at the debt. Then they can attack it. Maybe you have to get mad at your fat. It's your enemy, dragging you down, trying to kill you. Now attack it!

THE ENERGY BALANCE EQUATION

Where does the fat go when you lose weight dieting? Metabolic reactions convert it to energy, water, and carbon dioxide, which weigh less than fat. Most of your energy supply is used to fuel basic life-maintaining physiologic processes at rest, referred to as resting or basal metabolism.

Basal metabolic rate (BMR) is expressed as calories per kilogram of body weight per hour. Even at rest, a kilogram of muscle is much more metabolically active than a kilogram of fat tissue. Muscular lean people sitting quietly in a room are burning more calories than are fat people of the same weight sitting in the same room. If you think a slow metabolism is cause of your excess weight, you can increase your metabolic rate through strength training that builds new muscle (see chapter 10).

Energy not used for basal metabolism is either stored as fat or converted by the muscles to physical activity. Excess energy not used in resting metabolism or physical activity is stored as fat.

If you want to lose excess weight and keep it off, note that the energy you eat, minus the energy you burn in metabolism and activity, determines your change in body fat. This is the "energy balance equation."

Energy is measured in calories. For example, if you eat 2,000 calories of energy daily, but burn up 2,300 calories daily, you will have a negative energy balance and your fat stores will go down. That is, you lose weight. On the other hand, if you eat 2,500 calories but only burn up 2,300, you gain weight over time.

Overweight and obesity result—at least in part—from an imbalance between energy intake and expenditure.

Is it really that simple?

Gary Taubes is the foremost authority promoting the idea that fattening and obesity are caused by an imbalance—a disequilibrium—in the hormonal regulation of fat tissue. The energy balance equation is much less important in his view. Think of the transformation of a skinny 10-year-old girl into a voluptuous young woman. It's not over-eating that leads to curvaceous fat deposits, growth of mammary tissue, and increase in height; it's hormonal changes beyond her control.

The primary hormonal regulator of fat storage is insulin. Elevated insulin levels lead to storage of food energy as fat. *Carbohydrates* are the major cause of insulin secretion and, therefore, *make us fat* when eaten in excess. On top of that, hormone changes may slow down our activity levels, further contributing to weight gain.

Taubes outlines his theories in his brilliant book of 2007, *Good Calories, Bad Calories: Fats, Carbs, and the Controversial Science of Diet and Health*. In 2010, he produced a condensed version more digestible to the general public, *Why We Get Fat; and What to Do About It*.

His theory of overweight could explain my observation that it's frequently difficult for type 2 diabetics to lose weight, more so than for the non-diabetic, especially on moderate- and high-carb diets. They may be *resistant* to insulin's glucose–lowering action while remaining *sensitive* to insulin's fat-storing action.

143

Several scientific studies have found that people losing weight on very-low-carb ketogenic diets eat fewer calories than before they started the diet. They don't have to consciously restrict calorie consumption: it's an automatic result of low-carb, high-fat eating. The percentage of energy from protein may be higher, too. Protein- and fat-rich diets tend to be more satiating than low-fat calorie-restricted weight-loss diets. In other words, the low-carbers don't have as much hunger; they're more easily satiated. The reduction in hunger may be caused by lower insulin levels.

I have little doubt that the energy balance equation applies to us, at least to some degree. People who swear they can't lose weight on extreme low-calorie diets have been locked up (with consent) in university medical center metabolic wards with access to food strictly controlled by staff. Ancel Keys, of Mediterranean diet fame, did a famous experiment on this. On appropriate calorie-restricted diets, everyone loses weight. When an exercise program is added, they lose more weight.

Gary Taubes argues that "We don't get fat because we overeat; we overeat because we're getting fat." We need to think of obesity as a disorder of excess fat accumulation, then ask why the fat tissue isn't regulated properly. Dozens of enzymes and hormones—but especially insulin—are at play either depositing fat into tissue, or mobilizing the fat to be used as energy. It's an active process going on continuously. Any regulatory derangement that favors fat accumulation will *cause* gluttony (overeating) or sloth (inactivity). So it's not your fault.

FREE WILL

Are you able to restrict your carbohydrate consumption, reduce calorie intake, or increase your physical activity? It comes down to whether we have free will. Free will is the power, attributed especially to humans, of making free choices that are unconstrained by external circumstances or by an agency such as divine will.

Will is the mental faculty by which one chooses or decides upon a course of action; volition.

Willpower is the strength of will to carry out one's decisions, wishes, or plans.

If we don't have free will, you're wasting time trying to lose weight through diet modification; nothing will get your weight problem under control. Even liposuction and weight-reduction stomach surgery will fail in time if you are fated to be fat. The existence of free will is confirmed for me by my education in religion and philosophy, my intuition, and most prominently, by my experience. I have seen hundreds of my patients lose weight and keep it under control. I didn't do it for them. No other person, pill, or agency did it for them. They didn't achieve success by being passive victims of external circumstances. They cut back on carbohydrates or calories, or they increased activity levels through strength of will. *They* did it.

The beauty of very-low-carb and low-carb diets is that they make it easier to reduce calorie consumption. Why not take advantage of that?

You can enhance your willpower and commitment to losing weight by learning about:

145

- how your body needs various nutrients
- how your body stores excess energy intake as fat through the effect of insulin
- how your body can convert fat to energy as needed for physical activity and metabolism
- the adverse health effects of excess body fat
- the benefits of exercise

STARTING NEW HABITS

You already have a number of good habits that support your health and make your life more enjoyable, productive, and efficient. For example, you brush your teeth and bathe regularly, put away clean clothes in particular spots, pay bills on time, get up and go to work every day, wear your seat belt, put your keys or purse in one place when you get home, balance your checkbook periodically.

At one point, these habits took much more effort than they do now. But you decided they were the right thing to do, made them a priority, practiced them at first, made a conscious effort to perform them on schedule, and repeated them over time. All this required discipline. That's how good habits become part of your lifestyle, part of you. Over time, your habits require much less effort and hardly any thought. You just do it.

Your decision to lose fat permanently means that you must establish some new habits, such as reasonable food restriction. You've already demonstrated that you have self-discipline. The application of that discipline to new behaviors will support your commitment and willpower.

SUPPORTIVE SOCIAL SYSTEM

Success at any major endeavor is easier when you have a supportive social system. And make no mistake: losing a significant amount of weight and keeping it off long-term is a major endeavor.

Your mate, friends, co-workers, and relatives may be help or hinder your weight-loss effort. It will help if they:

- give you encouragement instead of criticism
- don't tempt you with taboo foods
- show respect for your commitment and will-power
- give you time to exercise
- go on a diet or exercise with you, if they are overweight or need exercise
- understand why there are no longer certain foods in the house
- appreciate the nutritious, sensible foods that are now in the house
- forgive and understand when you occasionally backslide
- gently remind you of your commitment when needed
- reward you with compliments as you make progress
- don't compare your physique unfavorably with supermodels or surgically-sculpted bodies
- don't get jealous when you lose weight and are more attractive and energetic

Your social support system can make or break your commitment and willpower. Ask them to help you; don't assume they know automatically what you need.

147

WEIGHT GOALS

Despite all the chatter about how to lose weight, few talk about how much should be lost.

If you're overweight, deciding how much you should lose is not as simple as it seems at first blush. I rarely have to tell a patient she's overweight. She knows it and has an intuitive sense of whether it's mild, moderate, or severe in degree. She's much less clear about how much weight she should lose. If it's any consolation, clinicians in the field aren't always sure either.

Four weight standards have been in common usage over the last couple decades:

1. Aesthetic Ideal Weights
2. USDA/HHS Healthy Weights
3. Realistic Weights
4. Body Mass Index

Aesthetic Ideal Weights are somewhat personal, although clearly influenced by culture. You know without much thought at what weight you look your best. Whether others agree with you, and whether you could realistically hope to reach that weight, are entirely different matters.

If your personal Aesthetic Ideal Weight matches the Hollywood hunk or "it girl" du jour, prepare for failure. Thespians and models want to be thin because the camera puts weight on them. Many of our beloved photogenic celebrities workout three hours daily with a personal trainer. On top of that, many visit plastic surgeons.

It may help if you find a friend with your type of body frame and height who looks "normal" and healthy to you. What does he or she weigh? I also suggest validation of your Aesthetic Ideal Weight by a trusted adviser. Now you've got something to shoot for.

In 1995, the U.S. Department of Agriculture and U.S. Department of Health and Human Services issued a chart of Suggested Healthy Weight ranges. By the turn of the century, the USDA/HHS's Dietary Guidelines for Americans had abandoned the Healthy Weight table, recommending the use of body mass index instead (discussed later).

A Realistic Weight goal is one that you have a reasonable expectation of achieving, accompanied by significant psychological or medical benefits. This standard is flexible. There is no weight chart to consult since your potential psychological or medical benefits are unique. These weights tend to be higher than the other benchmarks thus far reviewed.

The Realistic Weight concept accepts that you can feel better, look better, and have fewer medical problems while falling far short of the recommended "healthy" body mass index. Many of the illnesses caused or aggravated by being overweight (including diabetes and prediabetes) are improved significantly by loss of only five or 10 percent of body weight. The Realistic Weight concept admits the body cannot always be shaped at will: much of your shape and fat distribution are genetically determined. If all your blood relatives have big buttocks, thighs, and legs, you will also, although you do have some control over degree.

For many people, the Realistic Weight concept is helpful and valid, and prevents the discouragement felt when performance falls short of ideal. Let's not allow the perfect to be the enemy of the good. It's not realistic to expect a 40-year-old mother of three to weigh the same as a 17-year-old girl with no kids.

Body mass index (BMI) is your weight in kilograms divided by your height in meters squared (kg/m^2). To determine your BMI but skip the math, use an online calculator such as this one: http://advancedmediterraneandiet.com/bmicalcula tor.html.

From a health standpoint, BMIs between 18.5 and 24.9 are the best for people under 65–75 years old. About a third of the United States population is at this healthy weight. If you are 5-feet, 3-inches tall, your maximum healthy weight is 140 pounds (63.6 kg, BMI 24.9). If you are 5-feet, 9-inches tall, your maximum healthy weight is 169 pounds (76.8 kg, BMI 24.9).

BMIs between 25 and 29.9 designate "overweight" and accurately describe about 35 percent of the U.S. population. A BMI of 30 or higher defines "obesity" and indicates high risk for poor health. About 30 percent of U.S. adults are obese. At a BMI of 35 and above, rates of death and disease increase sharply.

The BMI concept is helpful to researchers and obesity clinicians, but the number doesn't mean much yet to the average person on the street, nor to many physicians. It should be used more widely. Know your BMI. If it's under 25, any excess fat you carry is unlikely to affect your health and longevity; your efforts to lose weight would be purely cosmetic.

If we look only at older Americans—65 to 75 years old—being overweight, but not obese, seems to prolong life on average. Longest life spans are seen in these older people with a body mass index between 25 and 30. These numbers, of course, apply only to groups of people defined by BMI, not to individuals. We have little data specific to people with diabetes.

So, how much weight should you lose?

As a medical man, I endorse the healthy BMI concept (BMI 18.5 to 24.9). If you have weight-related health issues such as diabetes or prediabetes, aim for a BMI of 18.5-24.9, with 25 to 30 as your fallback position. If you're over 65, consider a goal BMI between 25 and 30.

It's important to set a weight goal. If you don't know where you're going, you'll never get there.

CREATIVE VISUALIZATION

How will your life be different after you make a commitment and have the willpower to lose weight and keep it off permanently?

Odds are, you'll be more physically active than you are now. Exercise will be a habit, three to six days a week. Not necessarily vigorous exercise, perhaps just walking for 30 or 45 minutes, and strength training. It won't be a chore. It will be pleasant, if not fun. The exercise will make you more energetic, help you sleep better, and improve your self-esteem. Exercise doesn't help much with most weight loss efforts, but may be critical to avoidance of weight regain for many people.

I must tell you that I rarely see anyone lose a major amount of weight and keep it off without a regimen including regular physical activity. I wish that weren't the case, but that's the reality I've witnessed. Please don't think you'll be an exception; the odds are overwhelmingly against you. Plan on regular exercise being a part of your new lifestyle, especially after the initial weight loss.

Commitment and willpower will alter your relationship with food. You'll eat to live, rather than live to eat. You have important things to do with your life, dreams to pursue, and so little time left. If you have no long-range goals and are unclear about your purpose for living, you're certainly not alone. Why not consult a spiritual adviser such as a minister, priest, or rabbi for guidance?

Food is a necessary and enjoyable tool that helps you achieve your goals and fulfill your purpose by keeping you strong and healthy. Chronic overindulgence is a distraction. Carrying excess baggage impedes your progress on life's journey.

Your new relationship with food will involve two phases: 1) weight loss, and 2) maintenance of that loss.

During the weight-loss phase, you'll occasionally feel deprived due to carbohydrate restriction. Your willpower will be tested and sometimes broken. But you recover control and press on. You don't have to swear off all your favorite foods forever, just limit them. You'll learn to eat reasonable portions; eat until you're full, not stuffed. You eat real food that's readily available and good for everyone in the household. You don't have to sit there sipping your dinner out of a can while others at the table eat chicken, sautéed broccoli, and salad.

You're excited and enthusiastic at first, full of hope, particularly when you lose those first three or four pounds (1.5 to 2 kg). You're not expecting to lose six or 10 pounds (3 or 4 kg) every week as in the TV infomercials because you know those results are bogus or unsustainable. You're happy losing a half to one-and-a-half pounds (0.3 to 0.7 kg) weekly because you know the loss is fat, not water or intestinal contents. You've held a pound of butter (four sticks or 0.5 kg)) in your hand—that's what you've lost. And it's quite an accomplishment. The excitement wears off after three to six weeks, but it's easier to deal with since you knew it was coming. You focus on the long-term benefits and renew your commitment. It helps that you're now getting compliments from your friends and co-workers.

After much dedicated effort on your part, you finally attain your goal weight. You feel good about yourself. You take pride, justifiably, in your hard work, discipline, and willpower. You look better, sleep better, have more energy, and have rewarded yourself with some new clothes. Your blood sugars and hemoglobin A1c are much lower. But this is a critical juncture with risk—the risk of regaining fat and losing control of blood sugars. You must successfully navigate the transition to "maintenance phase," in which you confirm and solidify your weight loss achievement while preventing weight regain. This is the most puzzling, problematic, and frustrating area in the field of weight management. To some extent, you must chart your own course.

You understand how insulin not only lowers blood sugar levels, but also is a key hormone controlling the storage of fat. Any carbohydrates you eat will tend to raise both sugar levels and insulin levels (assuming your pancreas beta cells are not totally "burned out.") You therefore decide to go very slowly with re-introduction of additional carbs while transitioning from the Ketogenic to the Low-Carb Mediterranean Diet. Too many carbs, or the wrong kind, can wreck your hard-won success.

In your weight-loss phase, you had been converting 400–600 calories worth of fat into weightless energy every day. You didn't have to count calories, just carbs. Now that you've reached your goal weight and have the will to stay there, you have options. You can 1) start eating an extra 400–600 calories daily, 2) drastically reduce your physical activity so that you burn 400–600 calories less every day, 3) mix No. 1 and No. 2 such that you increase your current calorie budget by 400–600 calories, or 4) gradually add back more carbs (as in the LCMD) until you just start to regain fat weight, then reduce carbs a bit. No. 4 is the easiest.

In view of exercise's benefits (see next chapter), many successful losers choose to eat more food and continue or start an exercise program.

As long as you eat under 20–30 grams of carbohydrate daily, you won't have much appetite for more food calories. Eating additional carbs, however, will stimulate secretion of more insulin from many diabetic and prediabetic pancreas glands. The insulin, in turn, may further stimulate appetite and assist with storage of calories as body fat. That's why this is a critical stage in weight and glucose management.

At this point—the transition from weight loss to maintenance of weight loss—the natural inclination is to start eating more carbohydrates than you need. And you know what will happen. You'll need perhaps even more commitment and willpower to keep from slipping back into your old habits, into your lifestyle of the last 10 years. You vow to admit this reality: you can never again eat all the carbohydrates you want, whenever you want, over sustained periods of time. You look at a brownie, a candy bar, or a piece of apple pie, and you ask yourself, "Do I really want to walk an extra hour or jog an extra three miles today to burn off those calories? Do I want to risk the medical consequences of a blood sugar spike?"

You vow also to admit this reality: you're going to "fall off the wagon" occasionally and gain four, five, or more pounds (2 kg) of fat. Excessive carb consumption is likely to be the cause. But it's not the end of the world. You're not a failure. An extra five or eight pounds won't hurt you one bit, physically. But you draw the line, stand up straight, hold your head high, and simply return to your weight-loss program for a month or two. You've done it before and know you can do it again.

Changing your lifestyle is like breaking a horse. You're in for a rough ride and you're going to get thrown a few times. But you pick yourself up, dust yourself off, and climb back on. With time and persistence, you prevail.

10

Exercise

Exercise is overrated as a pathway to major
weight loss. Sure, a physically inactive young
man with only five or 10 pounds (2 to 4 kg) to
lose might be able to do it simply by starting an exercise program. That doesn't work nearly as well for
women. The problem is that exercise stimulates appetite, so any calories burned by exercise tend to be
counteracted by increased food consumption.

On the other hand, exercise is important for diabetics and prediabetics in two respects: 1) it helps in
avoidance of overweight, especially after weight loss,
and 2) it helps control blood sugar levels by improving insulin resistance, perhaps even bypassing it.
Let's look at exercise in general, first.

EXERCISE BENEFITS

As many as 250,000 deaths per year in the United States (approximately 12% of the total) are attributable to a lack of regular physical activity. We know now that regular physical activity can prevent a significant number of these deaths. Exercise induces metabolic changes that lessen the impact of, or prevent altogether, several major illnesses, such as high blood pressure, coronary artery disease, diabetes, and obesity. There are also psychological benefits. Even if you're just interested in looking better, awareness of exercise's other advantages can be motivational.

Exercise is defined as planned, structured, and repetitive bodily movement done to improve or maintain physical fitness.

Physical fitness is a set of attributes that relate to your ability to perform physical activity. These attributes include resting heart rate, blood pressure at rest and during exercise, lung capacity, body composition (weight in relation to height, percentage of body fat and muscle, bone structure), and aerobic power.

Aerobic power takes some explanation. Muscles perform their work by contracting, which shortens the muscles, pulling on attached tendons or bones. The resultant movement is physical activity. Muscle contraction requires energy, which is obtained from chemical reactions that use oxygen. Oxygen from the air we breathe is delivered to muscle tissue by the lungs, heart, and blood vessels. The ability of the cardiopulmonary system to transport oxygen from the atmosphere to the working muscles is called maximal oxygen uptake, or aerobic power. It's the primary factor limiting performance of muscular activity.

Aerobic power is commonly measured by having a person perform progressively more difficult exercise on a treadmill or bicycle to the point of exhaustion. The treadmill test starts at a walking pace and gets faster and steeper every few minutes. The longer the subject can last on the treadmill, the greater his aerobic power. A large aerobic power is one of the most reliable indicators of good physical fitness. It's cultivated through consistent, repetitive physical activity.

PHYSICAL FITNESS EFFECT ON DEATH RATES

Regular physical activity postpones death.

Higher levels of physical fitness are linked to lower rates of death primarily from cancer and cardiovascular disease (e.g., heart attacks and stroke). What's more, moving from a lower to a higher level of fitness also prolongs life, even for people over 60.

METABOLIC EFFECTS OF EXERCISE

Where does the fat go when you lose weight dieting? Chemical reactions convert it to energy, water, and carbon dioxide, which weigh less than the fat. Most of your energy supply is used to fuel basic life-maintaining physiologic processes at rest, referred to as resting or basal metabolism. Basal metabolic rate (BMR) is expressed as calories per kilogram of body weight per hour.

The major determinants of BMR are age, sex, and the body's relative proportions of muscle and fat. Heredity plays a lesser role. Energy not used for basal metabolism is either stored as fat or converted by the muscles to physical activity. Most of us use about 70 percent of our energy supply for basal metabolism and 30 percent for physical activity. Those who exercise regularly and vigorously may expend 40–60 percent of their calorie intake doing physical activity. Excess energy not used in resting metabolism or physical activity is stored as fat.

Insulin, remember, is the main hormone converting that excess energy into fat; and carbohydrates are the major cause of insulin release by the pancreas.

To some extent, overweight and obesity result from an imbalance between energy intake (food) and expenditure (exercise and basal metabolism). Excessive carbohydrate consumption in particular drives the imbalance towards overweight, via insulin's fat-storing properties.

In terms of losing weight, the most important metabolic effect of exercise is that it turns fat into weightless energy. We see that weekly on TV's "Biggest Loser" show; participants exercise a huge amount. Please be aware that conditions set up for the show are totally unrealistic for the vast majority of people.

Physical activity alone as a weight-loss method isn't very effective. But there are several other reasons to recommend exercise to those wishing to lose weight. Exercise counteracts the decrease in basal metabolic rate seen with calorie-restricted diets. In some folks, exercise temporarily reduces appetite (but others note the opposite effect). While caloric restriction during dieting can diminish your sense of energy and vitality, exercise typically does the opposite. Many dieters, especially those on low-calorie poorly designed diets, lose lean tissue (such as muscle and water) in addition to fat. This isn't desirable over the long run. Exercise counteracts the tendency to lose muscle mass while nevertheless modestly facilitating fat loss.

How much does exercise contribute to most successful weight-loss efforts? Only about 10 percent on average. The other 90 percent is from food restriction.

FOUNTAIN OF YOUTH

Regular exercise is a demonstrable "fountain of youth." Peak aerobic power (or fitness) naturally diminishes by 50 percent between young adulthood and age 65. In other words, as age advances even a light physical task becomes fatiguing if it is sustained over time. By the age of 75 or 80, many of us depend on others for help with the ordinary tasks of daily living, such as housecleaning and grocery shopping. Regular exercise increases fitness (aerobic power) by 15–20 percent in middle-aged and older men and women, the equivalent of a 10–20 year reduction in biological age! This prolongation of self-sufficiency improves quality of life.

HEART HEALTH

Exercise helps control multiple cardiac (heart attack) risk factors: obesity, high cholesterol, elevated blood pressure, high triglycerides, and diabetes. Regular aerobic activity tends to lower LDL cholesterol, the "bad cholesterol." Jogging 10 or 12 miles per week, or the equivalent amount of other exercise, increases HDL cholesterol ("good cholesterol") substantially. Exercise increases heart muscle efficiency and blood flow to the heart. For the person who has already had a heart attack, regular physi-

161

cal activity decreases the incidence of fatal recurrence by 20–30 percent and adds an extra two or three years of life, on average.

EFFECT ON DIABETES

Eighty-five percent of type 2 diabetics are overweight or obese. It's not just a random association. Obesity contributes heavily to most cases of type 2 diabetes, particularly in those predisposed by heredity. Insulin is the key that allows bloodstream sugar (glucose) into cells for utilization as energy, thus keeping blood sugar from reaching dangerously high levels. Overweight bodies produce plenty of insulin, often more than average. The problem in overweight diabetics is that the cells are no longer sensitive to insulin's effect. Weight loss and exercise independently return insulin sensitivity towards normal. Many diabetics can improve their condition through sensible exercise and weight management.

MISCELLANEOUS BENEFITS

In case you need more reasons to start or keep exercising, consider the following additional benefits: 1) enhanced immune function, 2) stronger bones, 3) preservation and improvement of flexibility, 4) lower blood pressure by 8–10 points, 5) diminished premenstrual bloating, breast tenderness, and mood changes, 6) reduced incidence of dementia, 7) less trouble with constipation, 7) better ability to handle stress, 8) less trouble with insomnia, 9) improved self-esteem, 10) enhanced sense of well-being, with less anxiety and depression, 11) higher perceived level of energy, and 12) prevention of weight regain.

People who lose fat weight but regain it cite lack of exercise as one explanation. One scientific study by

S. Kayman and associates looked at people who dropped 20 percent or more of their total weight, and the role of exercise in maintaining that loss. Two years after the initial weight loss, 90 percent of the successful loss-maintainers reported exercising regularly. Of those who regained their weight, only 34 percent were exercising.

EXERCISE RECOMMENDATIONS

Now that you know the health benefits of exercise, it's a little easier to understand those crazy people you see jogging at 6 a.m. in below-freezing weather. I'm sure you're ready to join them tomorrow morning. Right?

Here's some good news. Most people following both the Ketogenic and Low-Carb Mediterranean Diets are able to lose excess weight and improve glucose control without starting an exercise program. Many—but certainly not all—will be able to maintain a stable, reasonable weight and glucose control long-term without ongoing exercise. However, for the reasons already outlined, I recommend you start a physical activity program eventually.

I must warn you that athletic individuals who perform vigorous exercise should expect a deterioration in performance levels during the first three to four weeks of any very-low-carb ketogenic diet. The body needs that time to adjust to burning mostly fat for fuel rather than carbohydrate.

Also, competitive weight-lifters or other anaerobic athletes (e.g., sprinters) will be hampered by the low muscle glycogen stores that accompany ketogenic diets. They need more carbohydrates for high-level performance.

163

HOW MUCH EXERCISE?

All I'm asking you to do is aerobic activity, such as walk briskly (3–4 mph or 4.8–6.4 km/h) for 30 minutes most days of the week, and do some muscle-strengthening exercises three times a week. These recommendations are also consistent with the American Diabetes Association's Standards of Care–2011. This amount of exercise will get you most of the documented health benefits. It's OK if you want to wait until you've lost some of your excess weight, but I probably wouldn't.

Keep reading to find out if exercise would be a bad idea for you, depending on the presence of diabetic complications.

For the general public without diabetes, the U.S. Centers for Disease Control and Prevention recommends at least 150 minutes per week of moderate-intensity aerobic activity (e.g., brisk walking) and muscle-strengthening activity at least twice a week, OR 75 minutes per week of vigorous-intensity aerobic activity (e.g., running or jogging) plus muscle-strengthening activity at least twice a week. The muscle-strengthening activity should work all the major muscle groups: legs, hips, back, abdomen, chest, shoulders, arms.

Please note that you don't have to run marathons (26.2 miles) or compete in the Ironman Triathlon to earn the health benefits of exercise. However, if health promotion and disease prevention are your goals, plan on a lifetime commitment to regular physical activity.

STRENGTH TRAINING

What's "strength training"? It's also called muscle-strengthening activity, resistance training, weight training, and resistance exercise. Examples include lifting weights, work with resistance bands, digging, shoveling, yoga, push-ups, chin-ups, and other exercises that use your body weight or other loads for resistance.

Strength training three times a week increases your strength and endurance, allows you to sculpt your body to an extent, and counteracts the loss of lean body mass (muscle) so often seen during efforts to lose excess weight. It also helps maintain your functional abilities as you age. For example, it's a major chore for many 80-year-olds to climb a flight of stairs, carry in a bag of groceries from the car, or vacuum a house. Strength training helps maintain these abilities that youngsters take for granted.

According to the U.S. Centers for Disease Control and Prevention: "To gain health benefits, muscle-strengthening activities need to be done to the point where it's hard for you to do another repetition without help. A repetition is one complete movement of an activity, like lifting a weight or doing a sit-up. Try to do 8–12 repetitions per activity that count as 1 set. Try to do at least 1 set of muscle-strengthening activities, but to gain even more benefits, do 2 or 3 sets."

If this is starting to sound like Greek to you, consider instruction by a personal trainer at a local gym or health club. That's a good investment for anyone unfamiliar with strength training, in view of its great benefits and the potential harm or waste of time from doing it wrong. Alternatives to a personal

165

trainer would be help from an experienced friend or instructional DVD. If you're determined to go it alone, Internet resources may help, but be careful. Consider "Growing Stronger: Strength Training for Older Adults" (http://www.cdc.gov/physicalactivity/downloads/gr owing_stronger.pdf). Doug Robb's blog, HealthHabits, is a wonderful source of strength training advice (http://www.healthhabits.ca/). The Internet resources I've mentioned are not designed specifically for people with diabetes.

Current strength training techniques are much different than what you remember from high school 30 years ago—modern methods are better. Some of the latest research suggests that strength training may be even more beneficial than aerobic exercise.

AEROBIC ACTIVITY

What's "aerobic activity"? Just about anything that mostly makes you huff and puff. In other words, get short of breath to some degree. Examples are brisk walking, swimming, golf (pulling a cart or carrying clubs), lawn work, painting, home repair, racket sports and table tennis, house cleaning, leisurely canoeing, jogging, bicycling, jumping rope, and skiing. The possibilities are endless. A leisurely stroll in the shopping mall doesn't qualify, unless that makes you short of breath. Don't laugh: that *is* a workout for many who are obese.

But which aerobic physical activity is best? Glad you asked!

The most important criterion is that it be pleasant for you. If not outright fun, it should be often enjoyable and always tolerable.

Your exercise of choice should also be available year-round, affordable, safe, and utilize large muscle groups. The greater mass and number of muscles used, the more calories you will burn, which is important if you're trying to lose weight or prevent gain. Compare tennis playing with sitting in a chair squeezing a tennis ball repetitively. The tennis player burns calories much faster. Your largest muscles are in your legs, so consider walking, biking, many team sports, ski machines, jogging, treadmill, swimming, water aerobics, stationary cycling, stair-steppers, tennis, volleyball, roller-skating, rowing, jumping rope, and yard work.

Walking is "just what the doctor ordered" for many people. It's readily available, affordable, usually safe, and requires little instruction. If it's too hot, too cold, or rainy outside, you can do it in a mall, gymnasium, or health club.

Another option is instructional exercise DVDs, often featuring either a celebrity or prominent fitness trainer. Many of these programs require only a pair of sneakers and loose clothing. Others include the option of using inexpensive equipment, such as light hand-held weights.

If exercise videos sound appealing, consider one of these: Walk Away the Pounds—Walk Strong, by Leslie Sansone; Tighter Assets With Tamilee: Weight Loss & Cardio, by Tamilee Webb; Burn & Firm—Circuit Training, by Karen Voight; Minna Optimizer—Balanced Blend, by Minna Lessig; Personal Training System, by Denise Austin; Timesaver—Lift Weights to Lose Weight (volumes 1 & 2), Super Slimdown Circuit, and Functionally Fit—Peak Fat Burning, by Kathy Smith. Search for these titles at Amazon.com, where you can read reviews of them by actual users. Although many of these are designed for weight loss, you'll get a good workout even if you're at a healthy weight. Several of them also feature strength training.

Another fun option for indoor aerobic exercise is Dance Dance Revolution by Konami. Perhaps you've seen a version of this video game in an arcade. You must use a video game console, such as a PlayStation or Xbox, and the Dance Dance Revolution Controller along with your TV screen. The controller is a 32 inch by 36 inch (81 x 91 cm) floor pad partitioned into several large squares. The TV screen shows you which squares to step on in sequence as the music plays, and you rack up points for accurate timing and foot placement. If you enjoy moving to music, it's more fun than I can describe

The latest indoor computerized exercise gadgets are the Kinect for Microsoft's Xbox 360, the PlayStation Move, and Wii Fit. Check'em out.

MAKE IT A HABIT

The main objective at this point is to make regular physical activity a habit. Establishment of a habit requires frequent repetition over at least two or three months, regardless of the weather, whether you feel like it or not. Over time the chosen activity becomes part of your identity.

To avoid injury and burn out, begin your exercise program slowly and increase the intensity of your effort only every two or three weeks. Your body needs time to adjust to its new workload, but it will indeed adjust. Enhance your enjoyment with proper attire, equipment, and instruction, if needed. Use a portable radio or digital music system like an iPod or Zune if you tend to get bored exercising.

The "buddy system" works well for many of my patients: agree with a friend that you'll meet regularly for walking, jogging, whatever. If you know your buddy is counting on you to show up at the park at 7 a.m., it may be just the motivation you need to get you out of bed. Others just can't handle such regimentation and enjoy the flexibility and independence of solitary activity.

If you like to socialize, join a health club or sports team. Large cities have organized clubs that promote a wide range of physical activities. Find your niche.

Don't be afraid to try something new. Expect some disappointment and failed experiments. Learn and grow from adversity and failure. Put a lot of thought into your choice of activity. Avoid built-in barriers. If you live in Florida you won't have much opportunity for cross-country skiing. If joining a health club is a financial strain, walk instead. Perhaps pick different activities for cold and warm weather. Or do several types of exercise to avoid boredom.

In summary, formation of the exercise habit requires forethought, repetition, and commitment. You must schedule time for physical activity. Make it a priority. Hundreds of my couch potato patients have done it, and I'm sure you can, too. I've seen 40-year-old unathletic, uncoordinated barnacles start exercising and run marathons two years later. (A marathon is 26.2 miles or 42.2 km.)

MEDICAL CLEARANCE

To protect you from injury, I recommend that you obtain "medical clearance" from a personal physician before starting an exercise program. A physician is in the best position to determine if your plans are safe for you, thereby avoiding complications such as injury and death. Nevertheless, most adults can start a moderate-intensity exercise program with little risk. An example of moderate intensity would be walking briskly (3–4 mph or 4.8–6.4 km/h) for 30 minutes daily.

Men over 40 and women over 50 who anticipate a more vigorous program should consult a physician to ensure safety. The physician may well recommend diagnostic blood work, an electrocardiogram (heart electrical tracing), and an exercise stress test (often on a treadmill). The goal is not to generate fees for the doctor, but to find the occasional person for whom exercise will be dangerous, if not fatal. Those who drop dead at the start of a vigorous exercise program often have an undiagnosed heart condition, such as blockages in the arteries that supply the heart muscle. The doctor will also look for other dangerous undiagnosed "silent" conditions, such as leaky heart valves, hereditary heart conditions, aneurysms, extremely high blood pressure, and severe diabetes.

The American Diabetes Association's Standards of Care—2011 states that routine testing of all diabetics for heart artery blockages before an exercise program is not recommended; the doctor should use judgment case-by-case. Many diabetics (and their doctors) are unaware that they already have "silent" coronary artery disease (CAD). CAD is defined by blocked or clogged heart arteries, which reduced the blood flow to the hard-working heart muscle. Your heart pumps 100,000 times a day, every day, for years without rest. CAD raises the odds of fainting, heart attack, or sudden death during strenuous exercise. I recommend a cardiac stress test (or the equivalent) to all diabetics prior to moderate or vigorous exercise programs, particularly if over 40 years old. CAD can thus be diagnosed and treated before complications arise. Ask your personal physician for her opinion.

Regardless of age and diabetes, other folks who may benefit from a medical consultation before starting an exercise program include those with known high blood pressure, high cholesterol, joint problems (e.g., arthritis, degenerated discs), neurologic problems, poor circulation, lung disease, or any other significant chronic medical condition. Also be sure to check with a doctor first if you've been experiencing chest pains, palpitations, dizziness, fainting spells, headaches, frequent urination, or any unusual symptoms (particularly during exertion).

Physicians, physiatrists, physical therapists, and exercise physiologists can also be helpful in design of a safe, effective exercise program for those with established chronic medical conditions.

EXERCISE AND THE DIABETIC

METABOLIC EFFECTS

Physical activity offers multiple benefits for everybody and specific benefits for diabetics and prediabetics. Muscles doing *prolonged* exercise soak up sugar from the blood stream to use as an energy source, a process occurring independent of insulin's effect. On the other hand, blood sugar may rise *ear-*

ly in the course of an exercise session. Regular exercise increases your body's sensitivity to insulin, helping to overcome the insulin resistance phenomenon so often associated with diabetes, prediabetes, metabolic syndrome, and overweight. By these mechanisms, exercise aids control of high blood sugars.

A combination of strength training and aerobic exercise for 20 minutes a day—if done right—will lower hemoglobin A1c an average of 0.34% (absolute decrease). Doubling the activity to 40 minutes a day will lower it by 0.7 to 1%. These improvements are in the range of improvement seen with single diabetic medications. Admittedly, it's a lot easier to pop a pill than exercise; so that's what many people do.

HDL cholesterol (the good stuff) in diabetics averages 20 percent below that of non-diabetics. Higher HDL levels are better for your heart. Exercise is one of the few things we know will raise HDL levels, although, frankly, it takes a lot of exercise. Very-low-carb eating, by the way, also tends to raise HDL cholesterol.

All these benefits accrue even in the absence of weight loss.

WARNINGS AND PRECAUTIONS

Diabetic Retinopathy

Diabetics with retinopathy (an eye disease caused by diabetes) have an increased risk of retinal detachment and bleeding into the eyeball called vitreous hemorrhage. These can cause blindness. Vigorous aerobic or resistance training may increase the odds of these serious eye complications. Patients with retinopathy may not be able to safely participate. If you have any degree of retinopathy, avoid the straining and breath-holding that is so often done during weightlifting or other forms of resistance exercise. Vigorous aerobic exercise may also pose a risk. By all means, check with your ophthalmologist first. You don't want to experiment with your eyes.

Diabetic Feet and Peripheral Neuropathy

Diabetics are prone to foot ulcers, infections, and ingrown toenails, especially if peripheral neuropathy (numbness or loss of sensation) is present. Proper foot care, including frequent inspection, is more important than usual if a diabetic exercises with her feet. Daily inspection should include the soles and in-between the toes, looking for blisters, redness, calluses, cracks, scrapes, or breaks in the skin. See your physician or podiatrist for any abnormalities. Proper footwear is important (for example, don't crowd your toes). Dry feet should be treated with a moisturizer regularly. In cases of severe peripheral neuropathy, non-weight-bearing exercise (e.g., swimming or cycling) may be preferable. Discuss with your physician or podiatrist.

Hypoglycemia

Low blood sugars are a risk during exercise if you take diabetic medications in the following classes: insulins, sulfonylureas, meglitinides, and possibly thiazolidinediones and bromocriptine. Hypoglycemia is very uncommon with thiazolidinediones. Bromocriptine is so new (for diabetes) that we have little experience with it; hypoglycemia is probably rare or non-existent. See drug details in chapter four. Diabetics treated with diet alone or other medications

173

rarely have trouble with hypoglycemia during exercise.

Always check your blood sugar before an exercise session if you are at risk for hypoglycemia. Always have glucose tablets, such as Dextrotabs, available if you are at risk for hypoglycemia. Hold off on your exercise if your blood sugar is over 200 mg/dl (11.1 mmol/l) and you don't feel well, because exercise has the potential to raise blood sugar even further *early* in the course of an exercise session.

As an exercise session continues, active muscles may soak up bloodstream glucose as an energy source, leaving less circulating glucose available for other tissues such as your brain. Vigorous exercise can reduce blood sugar levels below 60 mg/dl (3.33 mmol/l), although it's rarely a problem in non-diabetics.

The degree of glucose removal from the bloodstream by exercising muscles depends on how much muscle is working, and how hard. Vigorous exercise by several large muscles will remove more glucose. Compare a long rowing race to a slow stroll around in the neighborhood. The rower is strenuously using large muscles in the legs, arms, and back. The rower will pull much more glucose out of circulation. Of course, other metabolic processes are working to put more glucose into circulation as exercising muscles remove it. Carbohydrate consumption and diabetic medications are going to affect this balance one way or the other.

If you are at risk for hypoglycemia, check your blood sugar before your exercise session. If under 90 mg/dl (5.0 mmol/l), eat a meal or chew some glucose tablets to prevent exercise-induced hypoglycemia. Re-test your blood sugar 30–60 minutes later, before you exercise, to be sure it's over 90 mg/dl (5.0 mmol/l). The peak effect of the glucose tablets will be 30–60 minutes later. If the exercise session is long or strenuous, you may need to chew glucose tablets every 15–30 minutes. If you don't have glucose tablets, keep a carbohydrate source with you or nearby in case you develop hypoglycemia during exercise.

Re-check your blood sugar 30–60 minutes after exercise since it may tend to go too low.

If you are at risk of hypoglycemia and performing moderately vigorous or strenuous exercise, you may need to check your blood sugar every 15–30 minutes during exercise sessions until you have established a predictable pattern. Reduce the frequency once you're convinced that hypoglycemia won't occur. Return to frequent blood sugar checks when your diet or exercise routine changes.

These general guidelines don't apply across the board to each and every diabetic. Our metabolisms are all different. The best way to see what effect diet and exercise will have on your glucose levels is to monitor them with your home glucose measuring device, especially if you are new to exercise or you work out vigorously. You can pause during your exercise routine and check a glucose level, particularly if you don't feel well. Carbohydrate or calorie restriction combined with a moderately strenuous or vigorous exercise program may necessitate a 50 percent or more reduction in your insulin, sulfonylurea, or meglitinide. Or the dosage may need to be reduced only on days of heavy workouts. Again, enlist the help of your personal physician, dietitian, diabetes nurse educator, and home glucose monitor.

175

Finally, insulin users should be aware that insulin injected over muscles that are about to be exercised may get faster absorption into the bloodstream. Blood sugar may then fall rapidly and too low. For example, injecting into the thigh and then going for a run may cause a more pronounced insulin effect compared to injection into the abdomen or arm.

Autonomic Neuropathy

This issue is pretty technical and pertains to function of automatic, unconscious body functions controlled by nerves. These reflexes can be abnormal, particularly in someone who's had diabetes for many years, and are called autonomic neuropathy. Take your heart rate, for example. It's there all the time, you don't have to think about it. If you run to catch a bus or climb two flights of stairs, your heart rate increases automatically to supply more blood to exercising muscles. If that automatic reflex doesn't work properly, exercise is more dangerous, possibly leading to passing out, dizziness, and poor exercise tolerance. Other automatic nerve systems control our body temperature regulation (exercise may overheat you), stomach emptying (your blood sugar may go too low), and blood pressure (it could drop too low). Only your doctor can tell for sure if you have autonomic neuropathy.

REALISTIC GOALS

Sustained physical activity requires that your heart pump blood to the lungs and then to the exercising muscles. The muscles extract oxygen, sugar, and other nutrients for use in chemical reactions that enable the muscle to keep moving (contracting). To say that someone is physically fit simply means that the heart easily pumps a large volume of blood and the muscles extract and use nutrients very efficiently. The heart, after all, is just a hollow muscle that pumps blood. If you stimulate your heart muscle through exercise, it will become more powerful and able to pump more blood. Regular sessions of physical activity increase the metabolic efficiency and power of your other muscles, too. There are various degrees of fitness, with professional and Olympic athletes at the extreme upper end.

GETTING STARTED

I have had otherwise healthy overweight patients so "out of shape" that walking 20 yards to the mailbox was a real chore. They were tired and panting when they got to the mailbox and had to rest a bit before returning to the house. These folks are habitually sedentary and dramatically overweight. But you need not feel too sorry for them. After starting and maintaining an exercise program, these unfit people achieve the greatest degree of improvement in fitness level. They make more progress, and faster, than those who begin with a greater level of fitness.

The way to achieve aerobic fitness is to regularly challenge your large muscles to perform sustained physical activity. "Regularly" means at least four days a week, if not daily. Left alone, your muscles don't want to do much other than just get you through your day comfortably, without effort or aching or cramps. You must challenge them to do more, work a bit harder, tolerate a little aching. You will know you are challenging them during exercise when you perceive that mild to moderate effort is required to keep the activity going. You should be mildly short of breath, perhaps even perspiring lightly, yet still able to converse. "Sustained" physical activity means at least 30 minutes in a day. Most people find it a better use of their time to exercise for 30 minutes continuously rather than break it up into five or 10 minutes here and there.

Discontinuous activity (e.g., 10 minutes thrice daily) probably is just as good. If you think about it, there are many easy ways to increase your discontinuous physical activity. Consider taking the stairs instead of the elevator, parking far from the supermarket or workplace doors, walking the golf course instead of riding a cart.

If you're starting out in poor shape, you won't be able to do 30 minutes of any exercise without adverse effects. Don't even try. The worst thing you could do at this point is injure yourself or have such a horrible experience that you give up entirely. Thirty minutes of daily activity is your goal to achieve over the next four to 12 months. Moderate to high levels of fitness will take you six to 24 months. The most important thing when getting started is to exercise at least a little, five to 10 minutes, on most days of the week. And don't overdo it in terms of intensity. Start low, go slow. After three months, exercise will be a habit. Prolongation of your exercise sessions will be easy as your amazing body responds gradually to the workload through the process called physical conditioning.

If walking 30 minutes daily is too hard for you at first, try walking just an extra 10 or 20 minutes daily. If you can do that but it's a bit of a strain, gradually (every two weeks) increase your walking time by five minutes daily until you are up to 30 minutes. Average walking pace is 2 mph (3.2 km/h). Once you can comfortably handle 30 minutes daily, the next step is to increase your walking pace to 3 or 4 mph (4.8–6.4 km/h) for the entire 30 minutes.

178

Four mph (6.4 km/h) is definitely a brisk walk. It's difficult for many people to sustain over 30 minutes until they work up to it gradually. This is often done by walking at two paces, normal and brisk, during an exercise session. You might walk five minutes at normal pace, then five minutes briskly, alternating every five minutes until the session is over. Every two to four weeks, you can increase the minutes of brisk pace and taper off the normal pace. You're able to do this easily because your level of fitness is increasing.

I'm asking you to walk briskly (3–4 mph or 4.8–6.4 km/h) for 30 minutes most days of the week. This brisk pace burns roughly 200 calories per session, in case you're wondering. If you eat a 400-calorie muffin, it provides enough energy for a one-hour brisk walk. If you don't burn the muffin calories as exercise or basal metabolism, they'll turn into body fat. (But you're not eating muffins anymore, are you?!)

If you prefer physical activity other than walking, the general rule is to start slowly and gradually increase your effort (intensity) until you're up to about 30 minutes of moderate-intensity exercise most days of the week. Start low, go slow.

IF YOU ARE MARKEDLY OBESE

The more overweight you are, the harder it will be to exercise. At some point even light exercise becomes impossible. Average-height women tipping the scales at about 280 pounds (127 kg) and men at 360 pounds (164 kg) aren't going to be able to jog around the block, much less run a marathon. These weights are 100 percent over ideal or healthy levels. An actual "exercise program" probably won't be possible until some weight is lost simply through very-low-carb eating, calorie restriction, or bariatric surgery. The initial exercise goal for you may just be to get moving through activities of daily living and perhaps brief walks and calisthenics while sitting in a chair.

Markedly obese people who aren't up to the afore-mentioned extreme weights can usually tolerate a low-intensity physical activity program. At 50 percent over ideal weight, an average-height woman of 210 pounds (95 kg) is carrying 70 excess pounds (32 kg) of fat. Her male counter-part lugs around 90 pounds (41 kg) of unnecessary fat. This weight burden causes dramatic breathlessness and fatigue upon exertion, and makes the joints and muscles more susceptible to aching and injury. If you're skinny, just imagine trying to walk or run a mile carrying a standard five-gallon (19 liter) water cooler bottle, which weighs only 43 pounds (19.5 kg) when full. The burden of excess fat makes it quite difficult to exercise.

If you're markedly obese, several tricks will enhance your exercise success. I want you to avoid injury, frustration, and burn out. Start with light activity for only 10 or 15 minutes, gradually increase session length (e.g., by two to four minutes every two to four weeks) and increase exercise intensity only after several months. Your joints and muscles may appreciate easy, low-impact exercises such as stationary cycling, walking, swimming, and pool calisthenics/water aerobics. You may also benefit from the advice of a personal fitness trainer arranged through a health club, gym, or YMCA/YWCA. Check out several health clubs before you join. Some of them are primarily meat markets for beautiful slender yuppies. You may feel more comfortable in a gym that welcomes and caters to overweight people.

Hospitals are increasingly developing fitness centers with obese orthopedic, heart, and diabetic patients in mind.

PEDOMETERS

A pedometer attached to your waistband may help motivate you by tracking total step count, distance traveled, and calories burned. Reliable pedometers cost $20 to $30 and are available at sporting goods stores, sports shoe stores, and via the Internet.

Consumer Reports magazine in February, 2009, reviewed pedometers and their #1 Best Buy recommendation was the Omron HJ 112, which you can clip to your belt or waistband, or carry in your purse. It's available for around $15–30 (U.S.). #2 was the Accusplit AE 170 XLG ($30–35), which I own and recommend. The Accusplit AE 170 may be just as good. The only difference I see is that you can enter your specific goals into the XLG.

The Omron HIP (HJ 150, $20) is also very popular and probably the simplest one to use of the three mentioned. The guys at Obesity Panacea blog (Peter Janiszewski and Travis Saunders, both Ph.D.s) recommend the Omron HJ-303 ($35), which you can carry in your pocket instead of clipped to your waistband.

Sedentary people walk 2,000–4,000 steps daily as they go about their lives. Your goal now is 8,000–10,000 daily steps. Ten-thousand steps covers about 5 miles. Appropriate comfortable shoes are well worth the money.

TARGET HEART RATE

One rough way to gauge whether you are working hard enough is to monitor your heart rate, also known as pulse. Subtract your age from 220. The result is your theoretical maximum heart rate in beats per minute. Your heart rate goal, or target, during sustained aerobic exercise is a pulse that is 60 to 80 percent of your theoretical maximum pulse. For example: maximum heart rate for a 40-year-old is 180 (220 - 40 = 180), so the target heart rate zone during exercise is between 108 and 144 (60 to 80 percent of 180). Exceeding the upper end of the target zone is usually too uncomfortable to be sustainable. Exercise heart rates below the target zone suggest you're not working hard enough to reap the full long-term benefits of aerobic exercise.

Here's how to determine your pulse. After five or 10 minutes of exercise, stop moving and place the tips of your first two fingers lightly over the pulse spot inside your wrist just below the base of your thumb. Count the pulsations for 15 seconds and multiply the number by four. The result is your pulse or heart rate. It will take some practice to find those pulsations coming from your radial artery. If you can't find it, ask a nurse or doctor for help.

Like all rules-of-thumb, this target heart rate zone isn't always an accurate gauge of cardiovascular workout intensity. For instance, it is of very little use in people taking drugs called beta blockers, which keep a lid on heart rate.

As you become more fit, you'll notice that you have to work harder to get your heart rate up to a certain level. This is a sure sign that your heart and muscles are responding to your challenge. You may also want to monitor your resting heart rate taken in the morning before you get out of bed. Unfit, sedentary people have resting pulses of 60 to 90. Athletes are more often in the 40s or low 50s. Their hearts have become more efficient and just don't need to beat as often to get the job done.

As you become more fit, you'll also notice that you have more energy overall and it's easier to move about and handle physical workloads. You'll feel more relaxed and have a sense of accomplishment. Expect these benefits eight to 12 weeks after starting a regular exercise program.

EXERCISE EQUIPMENT

You don't need to spend hundreds of dollars for new exercise equipment. Check Craig's List (or similar) and the classified ads of your newspaper for big discounts on "pre-owned" motorized treadmills, stationary bicycles, rowing machines, dumbbells, weight machines, and other devices. Avoid the exclusive abdominal muscle exercisers. Remember, you want to exercise the large muscles. You may have great "abs" but no one will know it if they're camouflaged behind three inches of fat.

EXERCISE WITH JOINT AND BACK PAIN

Painful lower limb joints and chronic or recurrent back pain are an exercise barrier to many people. Those affected should consult a physician for a diagnosis, treatment, and advice on appropriate physical activity. If the physician isn't sure about an exercise prescription, consultation with an orthopedist, physiatrist, or physical therapist should be helpful. Generally, weight-bearing on bad joints should be minimized by doing pool calisthenics, sta-

183

tionary cycling, swimming, etc. Use your imagination. Particularly bothersome joints may not tolerate exercise, if ever, until weight is lost by other method. Light to moderate exercise actually reduces the pain and disability of knee degenerative arthritis. The effect is modest and comes with a small risk of injury such as bone fracture, cartilage tears, arthritis flare, and soft tissue strain.

SUMMARY

Again, the goal is 30 minutes of brisk walking most days of the week, plus strength training three days a week. Walking faster or longer, and more vigorous types of exercise, might help you lose weight faster and achieve higher levels of fitness. But committing much more time and energy to exercise just isn't going to happen for many folks. Fortunately, most of the general health benefits of an active lifestyle are gained by a simple 30-minute daily brisk walk or similar aerobic exercise. Diabetics gain additional advantage over their condition by adding a strength training program.

Exercise isn't for everybody, and not everybody responds to exercise with good weight management and becoming shapelier. Your heredity limits your response to exercise to an uncertain extent. I challenge you to define your limits by putting your body through the paces. You may still be able to control your weight and blood sugars even if you don't exercise. If you can't manage regular physical activity during your period of weight loss, at least give it another chance as you move into your maintenance-of-weight-loss phase. Regular exercise is the single best predictor of successful long-term weight management.

11

Long-Term Maintenance

IT'S NOT JUST A BLOOD SUGAR ISSUE

As a diabetic or prediabetic trying to get and stay healthy, you need at least two other players on your healthcare team: a physician and a registered dietitian. Additionally, diabetes nurse educators can be quite helpful in teaching you to manage your condition. Other care team members may include physician assistants, nurse practitioners, pharmacists, and nutritionists.

Dietitians are particularly helpful consultants when diabetes is first diagnosed and periodically thereafter to answer food questions, check on compliance with diet recommendations, and to review new dietary guidelines. Unfortunately, a majority of dietitians still believe the out-dated idea that high-carbohydate eating is healthy for diabetics and others who have demonstrable difficulty processing carbs. Be sure the dietitian you choose supports a low-carb way of eating.

Most primary care physicians such as family physicians and internists are well-trained to co-manage diabetes with you. I chose the word "co-manage" carefully. It's not like you have appendicitis and can turn over all management to a surgeon. With diabetes, you have to do more work than your physician. Your doctor will review your home glucose records, adjust medications, periodically examine you, and check blood work. You need a doctor who will support, or at least tolerate, your low-carb way of eating.

An endocrinologist can be an invaluable team member, either as your main treating physician or as a consultant to your primary care physician. You should definitely see one if you are not close to the standard treatment goals (in a section to follow) after working with your primary care physician.

PERIODIC TESTS, TREATMENTS, AND GOALS

The American Diabetes Association (ADA) recommends the following items be done *yearly* (except as noted) in non-pregnant adults with type 2 diabetes. [Incidentally, I don't necessarily agree with all ADA guidelines.] ADA guidelines with supporting documentation are available free on the Internet (search for "Standards of Medical Care in Diabetes—2011"):

- Lipid profile (every two years if results are fine and stable)

- Comprehensive foot exam
- Screening test for distal symmetric polyneuropathy: pinprick, vibration, monofilament pressure sense
- Serum creatinine and estimate of glomerular filtration rate
- Test for albumin in the urine, such as measurement of albumin-to-creatinine ratio in a random spot urine specimen
- Comprehensive eye exam by an ophthalmologist (if exam is normal, every two or three years is acceptable)
- Hemoglobin A1c at least twice a year, but every three months if therapy has changed or glucose control is not at goal
- Flu shots

Additionally, the 2011 ADA guidelines recommend:

- Pneumococcal vaccination. "A one time *re*vaccination is recommended for individuals >64 years of age previously immunized when they were <65 years of age if the vaccine was administered >5 years ago." Also repeat the vaccination after five years for patients with nephrotic syndrome, chronic kidney disease, other immunocompromised states (poor ability to fight infection), or transplantation.
- Weight loss for all overweight diabetics. "For weight loss, either low-carbohydrate [under 130 g/day], low-fat calorie-restricted, or Mediterranean diets may be effective in the short-term (up to two years)." For those on low-carb diets, monitor lipids, kidney function, and protein consumption, and adjust diabetic drugs as needed. "The optimal macronutrient composition of weight loss diets has not been established." (Macronutrients are carbohydrates, proteins, and fats.)

- Limit alcohol to one (women) or two (men) drinks a day.
- Limit saturated fat to less than seven percent of calories.
- During initial diabetic exam, screen for peripheral arterial disease (poor circulation). Strongly consider calculation of the ankle-brachial index for those over 50 years of age; consider it for younger patients if they have risk factors for poor circulation.
- In the early stages of diabetic chronic kidney disease, reduce protein intake to 0.8-1.0 grams per kilogram of body weight. In later stages, reduce to 0.8 grams per kilogram of body weight.
- Those at risk for diabetes, including prediabetics, should aim for a) moderate weight loss (about seven percent of body weight) if overweight, through low-fat/reduced-calorie eating, b) exercise: 150 minutes per week of moderate-intensity aerobic activity.

Obviously, some of my dietary recommendations you've read in this book conflict with ADA guidelines. The experts assembled by the ADA to compose guidelines were well-intentioned, intelligent, and hard-working. The guidelines are supported by 395 scientific journal references. I greatly appreciate the expert panel's work. We've simply reached some different conclusions. By the same token, I'm sure the expert panel didn't have unanimous agreement on all the final recommendations. I invite you to review the dietary guidelines yourself, discuss with your personal physician, then decide where you stand.

GENERAL TREATMENT GOALS

The ADA suggests general therapeutic goals for adult non-pregnant type 2 diabetics:

- Fasting blood glucoses: 70 to 130 mg/dl (3.9 to 7.2 mmol/l)
- Peak glucoses one to two hours after start of meals: under 180 mg/dl (10 mmol/l)
- Hemoglobin A1C: under 7%
- Blood pressure: under 130/80 mmHg
- LDL cholesterol: under 100 mg/dl (2.6 mmol/l). (In established cardiovascular disease: <70 mg/dl or 1.8 mmol/l.)
- HDL cholesterol: over 40 mg/dl (1.0 mmol/l) for men and over 50 mg/dl (1.3 mmol/l) for women
- Triglycerides: under 150 mg/dl (1.7 mmol/l)

The American Association of Clinical Endocrinologists (AACE) in 2007 proposed somewhat "tighter" goals:

- Fasting blood glucoses: under 110 mg/dl (6.11 mmol/l)
- Peak glucoses 2 hours after start of meals: under 140 mg/dl (7.78 mmol/l)
- Hemoglobin A1C: under 6.5%

I outlined my goals—glucose levels and hemoglobin A1c—for my personal patients in chapter two.

The ADA reminds clinicians, and I'm sure the AACE guys agree, that diabetes control goals should be individualized, based on age and life expectancy of the patient, duration of diabetes, other diseases that are present, individual patient preferences, and whether the patient is able to easily recognize and deal with hypoglycemia. I agree completely. For in-

189

stance, there's not much reason to aim for blood sugars of 100 mg/dl (5.56 mmol/l) in a 79-year-old expected to die of lung cancer in four months. The goal is comfort and symptom relief, even if sugars are 220 mg/dl (12.2 mmol/l).

Admittedly, the aforementioned goals are difficult for many diabetics to achieve, but they are worth your effort in terms of avoiding long-term complications of diabetes. You will need to see your doctor every three to six months, and more often if your glucoses are not well-controlled or you have other medical issues.

IN CONCLUSION

Remember when you first found out you had diabetes or prediabetes? Maybe you knew just enough to be scared to death, with visions of amputations, endless needles, dialysis, and a life cut short.

You're moving in the right direction now!

This is an exciting time to have diabetes or prediabetes. We've come a long way since Dr. John Rollo's low-carb diet of 1797 and Banting and Best's discovery of insulin in 1921. As we learn more about underlying disease mechanisms, new therapies are being discovered by unrelenting scientists every few years. The pace of advancement is accelerating.

Diabetics today will not face the rates of amputation, blindness, kidney failure, and premature death seen too often in the past.

It can only get better.

ADDITIONAL RESOURCES

BOOKS

Bernstein, Richard. *Diabetes Solution: The Complete Guide to Achieving Normal Blood Sugars.* Little, Brown and Company (New York), 2007.

Hirsch, James. *Cheating Destiny: Living With Diabetes, America's Biggest Epidemic.* Houghton Mifflin Company (New York), 2006.

Kronenberg (editor), Henry, et al. *Williams Textbook of Endocrinology* (11th edition). Saunders Elsevier (Philadelphia), 2008.

Taubes, Gary. *Good Calories, Bad Calories: Fats, Carbs, and the Controversial Science of Diet and Health.* Knopf (New York), 2007.

Taubes, Gary. *Why We Get Fat: And What to Do About It.* Knopf (New York), 2011.

Vernon, Mary and Eberstein, Jacqueline. *Atkins Diabetes Revolution.* HarperCollins Publishers, Inc. (New York), 2004.

INTERNET

About.com: Type 2 Diabetes. Guide: Elizabeth Woolley. http://diabetes.about.com/

About.com: Low Carb Diets. Guide: Laura Dolson. http://lowcarbdiets.about.com/

Active Low-Carber Forums (free information and support) http://forum.lowcarber.org/

American Diabetes Association (conventional information and support)
http://www.diabetes.org

Bob Pedersen's blog at Diabetes Daily
http://www.diabetesdaily.com/pedersen

Calorie Count (support, nutritional analysis, tracking)
http://caloriecount.about.com/

Carb Wars Blog by Judy Barnes Baker
http://carbwars.blogspot.com/

Diabetes Daily (information and support)
http://www.diabetesdaily.com/

DARdreams (low-carb recipes)
http://dardreams.wordpress.com/

Cherise Shockley's blog at Diabetes Daily (type 1.5 diabetes or latent autoimmune diabetes in adults)
http://www.diabetesdaily.com/shockley

Diabetes Forums
http://www.diabetesforums.com

Diabetes Self-Management
http://www.diabetesselfmanagement.com/

Diabetes Update by Jenny Ruhl
http://diabetesupdate.blogspot.com/

Diabetes Mine by Amy Tenderich (mostly type 1)
http://www.diabetesmine.com/

Diabetic Mediterranean Diet Blog by Steve Parker, M.D.
http://diabeticmediterraneandiet.com/

dLife (education and support)
http://www.dlife.com/

FitDay (support, nutritional analysis, tracking)
http://fitday.com/

Fat Head by Tom Naughton (low-carb lifestyle)
http://www.fathead-movie.com/

Health Habits by Douglas Robb (fitness and weight management)
http://www.healthhabits.ca/

Healthy Low Carb Living by Amy Dungan
http://healthylowcarbliving.com/

Hold the Toast! by Dana Carpender (low-carb lifestyle)
http://holdthetoast.com/

Jimmy Moore's Livin' La Vida Low Carb Blog (renowned low-carb advocate)
http://livinlavidalowcarb.com/blog/

Low Carb Age by Frank Hagan (low-carb lifestyle news)
http://lowcarbage.com/

Low Carb Friends (free information and support)
http://lowcarbfriends.com/

MyDiabetesCentral.com (education and support)
http://healthcentral.com/diabetes/

Splendid Low-Carbing by Jennifer Eloff (low-carb recipes)
http://low-carb-news.blogspot.com/

Self/NutritionData (food education and nutrient database)
http://nutritiondata.self.com

The Blog of Michael R. Eades, M.D. (renowned low-carb advocate and co-author of *Protein Power*)
http://proteinpower.com/drmike/

Unrestricted Tastes on Restricted Diets: Distinctive Diabetic Recipes by Chef Barrae
http://chefbarrae.blogspot.com/

Valerie's Voice: For the Health of It, by Valerie Berkowitz (low-carb diet and lifestyle)
http://valerieberkowitz.wordpress.com/

WebMD's Diabetes Health Center (conventional diabetes information and support)
http://diabetes.webmd.com/

ANNOTATED BIBLIOGRAPHY

(alphabetical by lead author)

Albanese, Emiliano, et al. Dietary fish and meat intake and dementia in Latin America, China, and India: a 10/66 Dementia Research Group population-based study. *American Journal of Clinical Nutrition*, 90 (2009): 392-400. *Older adults in low- to middle-income countries have a lower risk of dementia if they regularly eat fish.*

Alhassan, S., et al. Dietary adherence and weight loss success among overweight women: results from the A TO Z weight loss study. *International Journal of Obesity* (London), 32 (2008): 985-991. *This study compared the weight loss of 311 overweight women on one of four diets: Atkins (low-carb), Ornish (very low fat, vegetarian), Learn (low-fat), and Zone (moderate carb restriction, high protein, moderate fat). Atkins was a bit better than the other diets, in terms of long-term (one year) weight loss. But within each diet group, some women lost 40–50 pounds (18–23 kg), whereas others gained over 10 pounds (4.5 kg). Authors' conclusion: "Regardless of assigned diet groups, 12-month weight change was greater in the most adherent compared to the least adherent tertiles. These results suggest that strategies to increase adherence may deserve more emphasis than the specific macronutrient composition of the weight loss diet itself in supporting successful weight loss."*

Accurso, A., et al. Dietary carbohydrate restriction in type 2 diabetes mellitus and metabolic syndrome: time for a critical appraisal. *Nutrition & Metabolism*, 9 (2008). PMID: 18397522. *One of the watershed reports that summarize the major features and benefits, based on 68 scientific references.*

Beasley, J., et al. Is protein intake associated with bone mineral density in young women? *American Journal of Clinical Nutrition*, 91, (2010): 1,311-1,316. *Contrary to accepted wisdom, high protein intake does not seem to be harmful to mineralization of bone. Mineralization of bone is important because higher bone mineral content generally translates to lower risk of fractures.*

Benedetti, Andrea, et al. Lifetime consumption of alcoholic beverages and risk of 13 types of cancer in men: results of a case-control study in Montreal. *Cancer Detection and Prevention*, 32 (2009): 352-362. *Canadians investigators did not find an association between wine consumption and cancer, although several other cancers were linked to alcohol.*

Boden, G., et al. Effect of a low-carbohydrate diet on appetite, blood glucose levels, and insulin resistance in obese patients with type 2 diabetes. *Annals of Internal Medicine*, 142 (2005): 403-411. *In these 10 obese diabetics, a low-carb diet spontaneously reduced calorie consumption from 3100 daily to 2200, accounting for the weight loss—1.65 kg (3.63 pounds) in 14 days. Blood sugar levels improved dramatically and insulin sensitivity improved by 75%.*

Buckland, Genevieve, et al. Adherence to a Mediterranean diet and risk of gastric adenocarcinoma within the European Prospective Investigation into Cancer and Nutrition (EPIC) cohort study. *American Journal of Clinical Nutrition*, December 9, 2009, Epub ahead of print. DOI: 10.3945/ajcn.2009.28209. *The first study to show protection by the Mediterranean diet against gastric cancer.*

Church, Timothy, et al. Effects of aerobic and resistance training on hemoglobin A1c levels in patients with type 2 diabetes: A randomized controlled trial. *Journal of the American Medical Association*, 304 (2010): 2,253-2,262. *Compared against resistance training and aerobic training by themselves, the best improvement in hemoglobin A1c was achieved with a combination of the two.*

Daly, M.E., et al. Short-term effects of severe dietary carbohydrate-restriction advice in Type 2 diabetes—a randomized controlled trial. *Diabetes Medicine*, 23 (2006): 15-20. *Compared with a low-fat/reduced-calorie diet, weight loss was much better in the low-carb group over three months, and HDL ratio improved.*

Dauchet, L., et al. Fruits, vegetables and coronary heart disease. *Nature Reviews Cardiology*, 6 (2009): 599-608. DOI: 1011038/nrcardio.2009.131. *Fruit and vegetable consumption does not seem to reduce the risk of heart attacks (coronary heart disease), according to French epidemiologists.*

Davis, Nichola, et al. Comparative study of the effects of a 1-year dietary intervention of a low-carbohydrate diet versus a low-fat diet on weight and glycemic control in type 2 diabetes. *Diabetes Care*, 32 (2009): 1,147-1,152. *The Atkins diet was superior—for weight loss and glycemic control—when measured at three months, when compliance by both groups was still probably fairly good. After one year, the only major difference they found was lower HDL cholesterol in the low-carb eaters.*

Elhayany, A., et al. A low carbohydrate Mediterranean diet improves cardiovascular risk factors and diabetes control among overweight patients with type 2 diabetes mellitus: a 1-year prospective randomized intervention study. *Diabetes, Obesity and Metabolism*, 12 (2010): 204-209. *In overweight type 2 diabetics, a low-carbohydrate Mediterranean diet improved HDL cholesterol levels and glucose control better than either the standard Mediterranean diet or American Diabetes Association diet, according to Israeli researchers.*

Esposito, Katherine, et al. Effects of a Mediterranean-style diet on the need for antihyperglycemic drug therapy in patients with newly diagnosed type 2 diabetes. *Annals of Internal Medicine*, 151 (2009): 306-314. *A low-carbohydrate Mediterranean diet dramatically reduced the need for diabetic drug therapy, compared to a low-fat American Heart Association diet. The Italian researchers also report that the Mediterranean dieters also lost more weight over the first two years of the study.*

197

Fortes, C., et al. A protective effect of the Mediterranean diet for cutaneous melanoma. *International Journal of Epidemiology*, 37 (2008): 1,018-1,029. *The first study to show protection against melanoma by the Mediterranean diet.*

Foster, Gary, et al. Weight and metabolic outcomes after 2 years on a low-carbohydrate versus low-fat diet: a randomized trial. *Annals of Internal Medicine*, 153 (2010): 147-157. *Dieters on low-fat and low-carb diets both lost the same amount of weight after two years. Both groups received intensive behavioral treatment, which may be the key to success for many. Low-carb eating was clearly superior in terms of increased HDL cholesterol, which may help prevent heart disease and stroke.*

Franco, O., et al. Associations of diabetes mellitus with total life expectancy and life expectancy with and without cardiovascular disease. *Archives of Internal Medicine*, 167 (2007), 1,145-1,151. *Compared to those in the cohort free of diabetes, having diabetes at age 50 more than doubled the risk of developing cardiovascular disease. Compared to those without diabetes, having both cardiovascular disease and diabetes approximately doubled the risk of dying. Compared to those without diabetes, women and men with diabetes at age 50 died seven or eight years earlier, on average.*

Fung, Teresa, et al. Low-carbohydrate diets and all-cause and cause-specific mortality: Two cohort studies. *Annals of Internal Medicine*, 153 (2011): 289-298. *"In our 2 cohorts of U.S. men and women who were followed for 20 to 26 years, we observed that the overall low-carbohydrate diet score was only weakly associated with all-cause mortality. However, a higher* animal *low-carbohydrate diet score was associated with higher all-cause and cancer mortality, whereas a higher* vegetable *low-carbohydrate score was associated with lower mortality, particularly cardiovascular disease mortality". The difference between the animal and vegetable low-carb diets was seen only by comparing extreme deciles of food consumption. The study is suggestive, but not definitive.*

George, Stephanie, et al. Fruit and vegetable intake and risk of cancer: a prospective cohort study. *American Journal of Clinical Nutrition*, 89 (2009): 347-353. *"Intake of fruit and vegetables was generally unrelated to total cancer incidence in this cohort."*

Giovannucci, E., et al. Diabetes and Cancer: A Consensus Report. *CA: A Cancer Journal for Clinicians*, 2010. DOI: 10.3322/caac.20078. *Type 2 diabetes is associated with higher incidence of several cancers: liver, pancreas, uterus, colo-rectal, breast, and bladder. On a brighter note, diabetics have lower risk of prostate cancer.*

German, J. Bruce, and Dillard, Cora J. Saturated fats: What dietary intake? *American Journal of Clinical Nutrition*, 80 (2004): 550-559. *"To date, no lower safe limit of specific saturated fatty acid intakes has been identified. This review summarizes research findings and observations on the disparate functions of saturated fatty acids and seeks to bring a more quantitative balance to the debate on dietary saturated fat. Whether a finite quantity of specific dietary saturated fatty acids actually benefits health is not yet known."*

Gu, Yian, et al. Food combination and Alzheimer Disease risk. *Archives of Neurology*, 67 (2010). Epub ahead of print. DOI: 10.1001/archneurol.2010.84. *A particular eating pattern does seem to lower the risk of Alzheimers Disease, the most common type of dementia. Manhattanites were significantly less likely to develop dementia if they had 1) higher consumption of salad dressing, nuts, tomatoes, fish, poultry, cruciferous vegetables, fruits, dark and green leafy vegetables, and 2) lower consumption of high-fat dairy products, red meat, organ meats, and butter. The study authors note similarities of this dietary pattern to the Mediterranean diet, long associated with lower risk of dementia. They also document the strong association of moderate alcohol consumption with lower dementia risk.*

Gutschall, Melissa, et al. A randomized behavioural trial targeting glycaemic index improves dietary, weight and metabolic outcomes in patients with type 2 diabetes. *Public Health and Nutrition*, 12(2009): 1,846-1,854. *Lowering glycemic index (GI) led to improved control of blood sugar,*

199

better insulin sensitivity, and weight loss in people with type 2 diabetes given group education sessions.

Haimoto, Hajime, et al. Effects of a low-carbohydrate diet on glycemic control in outpatients with severe type 2 diabetes. *Nutrition & Metabolism*, 6:21 (2009). DOI: 10.1186/1743-7075-6-21. *A low-carbohydrate diet is just as effective as insulin shots for people with severe type 2 diabetes, according to Japanese investigators. Five of the seven patients on sulfonylurea were able to stop the drug.*

Halton, Thomas, et al. Low-carbohydrate-diet score and the risk of coronary heart disease in women. *New England Journal of Medicine*, 355 (2006): 1,991-2,002. *"Our findings suggest that diets lower in carbohydrate and higher in protein and fat are not associated with increased risk of coronary heart disease in women."*

He, M., et al. Whole-grain, cereal fiber, bran, and germ Intake and the risks of all-cause and cardiovascular disease-specific mortality among women with type 2 diabetes mellitus. *Circulation*, 121 (2010): 2,162-2,168. *Whole grain and bran consumption are linked to reduced overall death rates and cardiovascular disease deaths in white women with type 2 diabetes. Whole grain and bran consumption may indeed protect against death and cardiovascular disease in diabetic white women, but the effect is by no means dramatic.*

Hession, M., et al. Systematic review of randomized controlled trials of low-carbohydrate vs. low-fat/low-calorie diets in the management of obesity and its comorbidities. *Obesity Reviews*, 10 (2009): 36-50. *More people dropped out of the low-fat diets, indicating a higher degree of satisfaction with low-carb. Low-carbohydrate/high-protein diets "are more effective at 6 months and are as effective, if not more, as low-fat diets in reducing weight and cardiovascular disease risk up to 1 year."*

Hooper, L., et al. Dietary fat intake and prevention of cardiovascular disease: systematic review. *British Medical Journal*, 322 (2001): 757-763. *"In this review we have tried to separate out whether changes in individual fatty acid fractions are responsible for any benefits to health (using the technique of meta-regression). The answers are not definitive, the data being too sparse to be convincing. We are left with a suggestion that less total fat or less of any individual fatty acid fraction in the diet is beneficial."*

Hu, Frank B. Are refined carbohydrates worse than saturated fats? *American Journal of Clinical Nutrition*, ePub ahead of print on April 21, 2010. DOI: 10.3945/ajcn.2010.29622. *Higher intake of refined carbohydrates is associated with coronary heart disease [at least in women]. Replacing saturated fat with high-glycemic-index carbs increased the risk of heart attack in a recent Danish study, while replacement with low-glycemic-index carbs trended the opposite direction. The key point of Dr. Hu's editorial is that all carbs are not equal when it comes to heart disease: high-glycemic-index carbs are the bad boys. Many of our beloved, highly processed carbs are in that gang.*

Hu, Frank. Diet and cardiovascular disease prevention: The need for a paradigm shift. *Journal of the American College of Cardiology*, 50 (2007): 22-24. *Dr. Hu de-emphasizes the original diet-heart hypothesis, noting instead that ". . . reducing dietary glycemic load should be made a top public health priority."*

Johnston, Carol, et al. Examination of the antiglycemic properties of vinegar in healthy adults. *Annals of Nutrition and Metabolism*, 56 (2010): 74-79. *Vinegar reduces blood sugar elevations after meals containing complex carbohydrates. Previous studies established that a single vinegar dose around mealtime lowers after-meal blood sugar levels by up to 50%. The most effective dose of vinegar was 10 g (about two teaspoons or 10 ml) of 5% acetic acid vinegar (either Heinz apple cider vinegar or Star Fine Foods raspberry vinegar). This equates to two tablespoons of vinaigrette dressing (two parts oil/1 part vinegar) as might be used on a salad.*

King, Dana E., et al. Adopting moderate alcohol consumption in middle age: Subsequent cardiovascular events. *American Journal of Medicine*, 121 (2008): 201-206. *The new moderate drinkers were 38% less likely than persistent nondrinkers to suffer a new cardiovascular event (P =*

0.008, which is a very strong association). Wine-only drinkers were 68% less likely than nondrinkers to suffer a cardiovascular event. The study authors cite four other studies that support a slight advantage to wine over other alcohol types.

Knopp, Robert and Retzlaff, Barbara. Saturated fat prevents coronary artery disease? An American paradox. [Editorial.] *American Journal of Clinical Nutrition*, 80 (2004): 1.102-1.103. *"In conclusion, the hypothesis-generating report of Mozaffarian et al (2004) draws attention to the different effects of diet on lipoprotein physiology and cardiovascular disease risk. These effects include the paradox that a high-fat, high–saturated fat diet is associated with diminished coronary artery disease progression in women with the metabolic syndrome, a condition that is epidemic in the United States. This paradox presents a challenge to differentiate the effects of dietary fat on lipoproteins and cardiovascular disease risk in men and women, in the different lipid disorders, and in the metabolic syndrome."*

Krebs, N., et al. Efficacy and safety of a high protein, low carbohydrate diet for weight loss in severely obese adolescents. *The Journal of Pediatrics*, 157 (2010): 252-258. *High-protein, low-carbohydrate diets are safe and effective for severely obese adolescent, according to University of Colorado researchers.*

Kondo, Toomoo, et al. Vinegar intake reduces body weight, body fat mass, and serum triglyceride levels in obese Japanese subjects. *Bioscience, Biotechnology, and Biochemistry*, 73 (2009): 1,837-1,843. *Japanese researchers recently documented that daily vinegar reduces body weight, fat mass, and triglycerides in overweight Japanese adults. By the end of this 12-week study, weight had decreased by 1-2 kg (2.2 to 4.4 pounds) in the vinegar drinkers, with 30 ml of vinegar a bit more effective than lower doses. Vinaigrettes are combinations of olive oil and vinegar, often with various spices added. If you eat a salad twice a day, it would be easy to add 15 ml (1 tbsp) of vinegar to your diet daily.*

Malik, V., et al. Sugar-sweetened beverages, obesity, type 2 diabetes mellitus, and cardiovascular disease risk. *Circulation*, 121 (1010): 1,356-1,364. *Sugar-sweetened beverages may cause type 2 diabetes and cardiovascular disease—separate from their effect on obesity—via high glycemic load and increased fructose metabolism, in turn leading to insulin resistance, inflammation, pancreas beta cell impairment, high blood pressure, visceral fat build-up, and adverse effects on blood lipids.*

Mellen, P.B, et al. Whole grain intake and cardiovascular disease: a meta-analysis. *Nutrition, Metabolism and Cardiovascular Disease*, 18 (2008): 283-290. *Whole grain consumption is associated with a 21% reduction in cardiovascular disease when compared to minimal whole grain intake. The effective dose seems to be 2.5 servings a day. Disease events included heart disease, strokes, and fatal cardiovascular disease. The lower risk was similar in degree whether the focus was on heart disease, stroke, or cardiovascular death. Refined grain consumption was not associated with cardiovascular disease events.*

Mente, Andrew, et al. A Systematic Review of the Evidence Supporting a Causal Link Between Dietary Factors and Coronary Heart Disease. *Archives of Internal Medicine*, 169 (2009): 659-669. *The authors found insufficient evidence linking coronary heart disease to consumption of total fat, saturated fat, and polyunsaturated fat.*

Mozaffarian, Darius, et al. Dietary fats, carbohydrate, and progression of coronary atherosclerosis in postmenopausal women. *American Journal of Clinical Nutrition*, 80 (2004): 1,175-1,184. *"In postmenopausal women with relatively low total fat intake, a greater saturated fat intake is associated with less progression of coronary atherosclerosis, whereas carbohydrate intake is associated with a greater progression."*

Nield, L., et al. Dietary advice for treatment of type 2 diabetes mellitus in adults. Cochrane Database of Systematic Reviews 2007, Issue 3. Art. No.: CD004097. DOI: 10.1002/14651858.CD004097.pub4. *Reviewers looked at low-fat/high-carb diets, high-fat/low-carb diets, low-calorie diets, very-low-calorie diets, and modified fat diets. "There* are no high quality data on the efficacy of the dietary treatment of type 2 diabetes....There is an urgent need for well-designed studies which examine a range of interventions...."

Nielsen, Jörgen and Joensson, Eva. Low-carbohydrate diet in type 2 diabetes: stable improvement of body weight and glycemic control during 44 months follow-up. *Nutrition & Metabolism*, 5 (2008). DOI: 10.1186/1743-7075-5-14. *Obese people with type 2 diabetes following a 20% carbohydrate diet demonstrated sustained improvement in weight and blood glucose control, according to Swedish physicians. Proportions of carbohydrates, fat, and protein were 20%, 50%, and 30% respectively. Total daily carbs were 80-90 g. Hemoglobin A1c, a measure of diabetes control, fell from 8% to 6.8%. These doctors had previously demonstrated that a 20% carbohydrate diet was superior to a low-fat/55-60% carb diet in obese diabetes patients over six months.*

Oh, K., et al. Dietary fat intake and risk of coronary heart disease in women: 20 years of follow-up of the Nurses' Health Study. *American Journal of Epidemiology*, 161 (2005): 672-679. *Total saturated fat consumption are not even mentioned in the abstract. "Intakes of saturated fat and monounsaturated fat were not statistically significant predictors of coronary heart disease when adjusted for nondietary and dietary risk factors." "Intakes of total fat, saturated fat, and monounsaturated fat had no clear relation to coronary heart disease regardless of age group." Trans-fats and lower consumption of polyunsaturated fats were linked to higher risk of coronary heart disease.*

O'Riordan, Michael. Dieting by DNA? Popular diets work best by genotype, research shows. *HeartWire by TheHeart.Org*, March 8, 2010. *Dieters with particular genetic make-up respond better or worse to specific types of weight-loss diets, suggest researchers who presented data at the 2010 Cardiovascular Disease Epidemiology and Prevention / Nutrition, Physical Activity, and Metabolism conference.*

Parikh, Parin, et al. Diets and cardiovascular disease: an evidence-based assessment. *Journal of the American Col-*

lege of Cardiology, 45 (2005): 1,379-1,387. *"The Mediterranean Diet has been shown to be cardioprotective in both prevention of sudden cardiac death and secondary prevention." "The scientific community has also begun to question the low-fat diet-heart hypothesis." "Although none of the reviewed diets are independently perfect for weight loss and cardiovascular health, an optimal diet can be extracted from this review. Specifically, such a diet would encourage: 1) decreased carbohydrate intake, especially of refined and high-glycemic-index carbohydrates; 2) increased consumption of fruits, vegetables, and whole grains; 3) increased intake of polyunsaturated fats by increasing consumption of plant oils and fish; 4) and moderate intake of low-fat dairy products and nuts." Note: no mention of cholesterol, saturated fat, or total fat.*

Parker, Steve. Health benefits of the Mediterranean diet. Advanced Mediterranean Diet Blog, July 29, 2010. Accessed October 20, 2010. http://advancedmediterraneandiet.com/blog/2010/07/29/documented-health-benefits-of-the-mediterranean-diet-or-whats-the-healthiest-diet/. *Comprehensive list of Mediterranean diet health benefits with supporting references.*

Parker, Steve. Are saturated fats really all that bad? Advanced Mediterranean Diet Blog, July 6, 2009. Accessed October 20, 2010. http://advancedmediterraneandiet.com/blog/2009/07/06/are-saturated-fats-really-all-that-bad/. *Comprehensive list of scientific references supporting the idea that dietary saturated and total fat are unrelated to cardiovascular disease.*

Perez-Jimenez, Jara and Saura-Calixto, Fulgencio. Grape products and cardiovascular disease risk factors. *Nutrition Research Reviews*, 21 (2008): 158-173. *Grape products favorably affect four risk factors for heart disease.*

Perez-Guisado, J., Munoz-Serrano, A., and Alonso-Moraga, A. Spanish Ketogenic Mediterranean diet: a healthy cardiovascular diet for weight loss. *Nutrition Journal*, 7, (2008). DOI:10.1186/1475-2891-7-30. *"The Spanish Ketogenic Mediterranean Diet is a safe and effective way of losing weight, promoting non-atherogenic lipid pro-*

files, lowering blood pressure and improving fasting blood glucose levels."

Ramel, A., et al. Consumption of cod and weight loss in young overweight and obese adults on an energy reduced diet for 8-weeks. *Nutrition, Metabolism and Cardiovascular Diseases*, 19 (2009): 690-696. *Five servings of cod per week led to loss of an extra 3.7 pounds (1.7 kg) over eight weeks, compared to a group not eating seafood.*

Ravsnskov, U. Hypothesis out-of-date. The diet-heart idea. *Journal of Clinical Epidemiology*, 55 (2002): 1,057-1,063. *"An almost endless number of observations and experiments have effectively falsified the hypothesis that dietary cholesterol and fats, and a high cholesterol level play a role in the causation of atherosclerosis and cardiovascular disease. The hypothesis is maintained because allegedly supportive, but insignificant findings, are inflated, and because most contradictory results are misinterpreted, misquoted or ignored."*

Ravnskov, U, et al. Studies of dietary fat and heart disease. *Science*, 295 (2002): 1,464-1,465. *Similar to the author's 2002 article above, in Journal of Clinical Epidemiology.*

Ravnskov, U. The questionable role of saturated and polyunsaturated fatty acids in cardiovascular disease. *Journal of Clinical Epidemiology*, 51 (1998): 443-460. *The author reviews available clinical evidence as of the late 1990s, questioning the harmful effect of dietary saturated fatty acids and the protective effect of dietary polyunsaturated fatty acids on atherosclerosis and cardiovascular disease.*

Razquin, C., et al. A 3 year follow-up of a Mediterranean diet rich in virgin olive oil is associated with high plasma antioxidant capacity and reduced body weight gain. *European Journal of Clinical Nutrition*, 63 (2009): 1,387-1,393. *The Mediterranean diet with supplemented with virgin olive oil may help you keep weight under control, and the enhanced antioxidant capacity may contribute to the well-documented health benefits of the diet.*

Sabaté, Joan and Ang, Yen. Nuts and health outcomes: New epidemiologic evidence. *American Journal of Clinical Nutrition*, 89 (2009): 1,643S-1,648S. *Nut consumption is strongly linked to reduced coronary heart disease, with less rigorous evidence for several other health benefits. Frequent and long-term nut consumption is linked to: reduced coronary heart disease (heart attacks, for example), reduced risk of diabetes in women (in men, who knows?), less gallstone disease in both sexes, lower body weight and lower risk of obesity and weight gain. The heart-protective dose of nuts is three to five 1-ounce servings a week.*

Salas-Salvado, Jordi, et al. Effect of a Mediterranean Diet Supplemented With Nuts on Metabolic Syndrome Status: One-Year Results of the PREDIMED Randomized Trial. *Archives of Internal Medicine*, 168 (2008): 2,449-2,458. *After one year of intervention, the prevalence of metabolic syndrome was reduced by 14% in the Mediterranean diet plus nuts group compared to the control, low-fat diet group.*

Samaha, F., et al. A low-carbohydrate as compared with a low-fat diet in severe obesity. *New England Journal of Medicine*, 348 (2003): 2,074-2,081. *Forty percent of subjects had diabetes. The low-carb Atkins-style group lost 5.8 kg (13 lb); the low-fat group lost 1.9 kg (4 lb). White subjects lost more weight than blacks: 13 versus 5 kg (29 versus 11 lb). Total cholesterol, HDL cholesterol, and LDL cholesterol levels did not change significantly within or between groups. [HDL usually rises on a low-carb diet.] Triglycerides fell 20% in the low-carb group and 4% in the other group. For subjects with diabetes, glucose levels fell 26 mg/dl in the low-carb group compared to 5 mg/dl in the low-fat group. Uric acid levels didn't change in either group. [Elevated uric acid levels can cause gout.] No significant adverse reactions attributable to the diets were recorded in either group. Glycosylated hemoglobin fell from 7.8 to 7.2% in the low-carb group, with no change in the low-fat group.*

SanGiovanni, J.P., et al. Long-chain polyunsaturated fatty acid intake and 12-y incidence of neovascular age-related macular degeneration and central geographic atrophy: AREDS report 30, a prospective cohort study from the

Age-Related Eye Disease Study. *American Journal of Clinical Nutrition*, 90 (2009): 1,601-1,607. *Age-related macular degeneration is the leading cause of blindness in Americans over 65. Impaired vision precedes blindness. This study linked consumption of omega-3 fatty acids (as in cold-water fatty fish) with 30% lower risk of developing macular degeneration.*

Shai, Iris, et al. Weight Loss with a Low-Carbohydrate, Mediterranean, or Low-Fat Diet. *New England Journal of Medicine*, 359 (2008): 229-241. *The researchers conclude that "Mediterranean and low-carbohydrate diets may be effective alternatives to low-fat diets. The more favorable effects on lipids (with the low-carbohydrate diet) and on glycemic control (with the Mediterranean diet) suggest that personal preferences and metabolic considerations might inform individualized tailoring of dietary interventions."*

Shai, Iris, et al. Glycemic effects of moderate alcohol intake among patients with type 2 diabetes: A multicenter, randomized, clinical intervention trial. *Diabetes Care*, 30 (2007): 3,011-3,016. *Wine consumption lowered fasting blood sugar levels by 15% in type 2 diabetics in Israel who had previously not been habitual drinkers.*

Sieri, Sabina, et al. Dietary glycemic load and index and risk of coronary heart disease in a large Italian cohort. The EPICOR study. *Archives of Internal Medicine*, 170 (2010): 640-647. *Italian women with the highest consumption of carbohydrates had twice the incidence of coronary heart disease compared to those with lowest consumption. No such relationship was seen in men.*

Sievenpiper, J.L., et al. Effect of non-oil-seed pulses on glycaemic control: a systematic review and meta-analysis of randomised controlled experimental trials in people with and without diabetes. *Diabetologia*, 52 (2009): 1,479-1,495. *Beans and peas improve control of blood sugar in diabetics and others, according to these Canadian researchers. The effect is modest. Pulse given alone or as part of a high-fiber or low-glycemic index diet improved markers of glucose control, such as fasting blood sugar and hemoglobin A1c. The absolute improvement in HgbA1c was around 0.5%. Effects in healthy non-diabetics were less dramatic or non-existent.*

Siri-Tarino, Patty, et al. Meta-analysis of prospective cohort studies evaluating the association of saturated fat with cardiovascular disease. *American Journal of Clinical Nutrition*, January 13, 2010. doi:10.3945/ajcn.2009.27725. *"A meta-analysis of prospective epidemiologic studies showed that there is no significant evidence for concluding that dietary saturated fat is associated with an increased risk of coronary heart disease or cardiovascular disease."*

Skeaff, C. Murray and Miller, Jody. Dietary fat and coronary heart disease: Summary of evidence from prospective cohort and randomised controlled trials. *Annals of Nutrition and Metabolism*, 55 (2009): 173-201. *"The available evidence from cohort and randomised controlled trials is unsatisfactory and unreliable to make judgment about and substantiate the effects of dietary fat on risk of CHD."*

Sluijs, I., et al. Carbohydrate quantity and quality and risk of type 2 diabetes in the European Prospective Investigation into Cancer and Nutrition-Netherlands (EPIC-NL) study. *The American Journal of Clinical Nutrition*, 92, (2010): 905-911. *High consumption of carbohydrates, high-glycemic-index eating, and high-glycemic-load eating increases the risk of developing diabetes. High fiber consumption, on the other hand, seems to protect against diabetes.*

Sofi, Francesco, et al. Accruing evidence about benefits of adherence to the Mediterranean diet on health: an updated systematic review and meta-analysis. American Journal of Clinical Nutrition, ePub ahead of print, September 1, 2010. doi: 10.3945/ajcn.2010.29673. *This expands Sofi and associates' 2008 study to include Mediterranean diet's protection against mild cognitive impairment and stroke.*

Sofi, Francesco, et al. Adherence to Mediterranean diet and health status: Meta-analysis. British Medical Journal, 337; a1344. Published online September 11, 2008. DOI:10.1136/bmj.a1344. *The Mediterranean diet reduces overall deaths, cardiovascular deaths, and incidence of Parkinsons disease and Alzheimers disease.*

Taubes, G. The soft science of dietary fat. *Science*, 291 (2001): 2535-2541. *One of the first popular press articles questioning the role of dietary fat in heart and vascular disease.*

Vernon, M., et al. Clinical experience of a carbohydrate-restricted diet: Effect on diabetes mellitus. *Metabolic Syndrome and Related Disorders*, 1 (2003): 233-238. *This groundbreaking study demonstrated that diabetics could use an Atkins-style diet safely and effectively in a primary care setting.*

Weinberg, W.C. The Diet-Heart Hypothesis: a critique. *Journal of the American College of Cardiology*, 43 (2004): 731-733. *"The low-fat "diet–heart hypothesis" has been controversial for nearly 100 years. The low-fat–high-carbohydrate diet, promulgated vigorously by the National Cholesterol Education Program, National Institutes of Health, and American Heart Association since the Lipid Research Clinics-Primary Prevention Program in 1984, and earlier by the U.S. Department of Agriculture food pyramid, may well have played an unintended role in the current epidemics of obesity, lipid abnormalities, type II diabetes, and metabolic syndromes. This diet can no longer be defended by appeal to the authority of prestigious medical organizations or by rejecting clinical experience and a growing medical literature suggesting that the much-maligned low-carbohydrate–high-protein diet may have a salutary effect on the epidemics in question."*

Westman, Eric, et al. The effect of a low-carbohydrate, ketogenic diet versus a low-glycemic index diet on glycemic control in type 2 diabetes mellitus. *Nutrition & Metabolism*, 5 (2008). DOI: 10.1186/1743-7075-5-36. *Duke University (U.S.) researchers demonstrated better improvement and reversal of type 2 diabetes with an Atkins-style diet, compared to a low-glycemic index reduced-calorie diet.*

Yancy, William, et al. A low-carbohydrate, ketogenic diet to treat type 2 diabetes [in men]. *Nutrition & Metabolism*, 2:34 (2005). DOI: 10.1186/1743-7075-2-34. *A low-carb* ketogenic diet in patients with type 2 diabetes was so effective that diabetes medications were reduced or discontinued in most patients. *The authors recommend that similar dieters be under close medical supervision or capable of adjusting their own medication, because the diet lowers blood sugar dramatically.*

Yancy, W., et al. A pilot trial of a low-carbohydrate ketogenic diet in patients with type 2 diabetes. *Metabolic Syndrome and Related Disorders*, 1 (2003): 239-244. *This pioneering study used an Atkins Induction-style diet with less than 20 grams of carbohydrate daily.*

Yusuf, S., et al. Effect of potentially modifiable risk factors associated with myocardial infarction in 52 countries (the INTERHEART study): case-control study. *Lancet*, 364 (2004): 937-952. *Consumption of cholesterol, total fat, and saturated fat are not even mentioned in the abstract of this article. ApoB/ApoA1 ratio was a risk factor for heart attack, so dietary saturated fat may play a role if it affects this ratio.*

Zarraga, Ignatius, and Schwartz, Ernst. Impact of dietary patterns and interventions on cardiovascular health. *Circulation*, 114 (2006): 961-973. *"Numerous studies have been conducted to help provide dietary recommendations for optimal cardiovascular health. The most compelling data appear to come from trials that tested diets rich in fruits, vegetables, monounsaturated fatty acids, and polyunsaturated fatty acids, particularly the omega-3 polyunsaturated fatty acids. In addition, some degree of balance among various food groups appears to be a more sustainable behavioral practice than extreme restriction of a particular food group."*

INDEX

A

Acarbose, 33
Active Low-Carbers
    Forum, 120
Actos, 52
Aerobic activity, 166
Aerobic power, 158
Aging, 161
Alcohol
    alternatives to wine, 77
    warning, 74
Alpha-glucosidase
    inhibitors, 33
American Association of
    Clinical
    Endocrinologists, 189
American Diabetes
    Association, 186
Amylin, 48
Avandia, 52

B

Banting, Frederick, 20
Basal metabolic rate, 159
Bernstein, Richard K.,
    10, 14
Best, Charles, 20
Biggest Loser, 160
Bile acid sequestrant, 36
Biquanide, 46

Blood pressure, low, 124
Blood sugar. *See* Glucose,
    blood
Body mass index, 150
Bromocriptine, 34
Byetta, 39

C

Calorie Count website,
    131
Carbohydrates
    average U.S. consumption,
        56
    definition of low-carb diet,
        56
    definition of very-low-carb
        diet, 56
    main sources, 56
    metabolism in diabetes, 18
    normal metabolism, 16
Carpender, Dana, 121
Centrum, 78
Cheating, 126
Chef Barrae, 120
Coffee, 78
Colesevelam, 36
Condiments, 77
Constipation, 123
Cookbooks, general, 134
Cookbooks, low-carb, 120
Cycloset, 34

D

Daily log, 130
Dancel, Jean-Francois, 10
DAR, 121
Diabetes
  complications, 11, 15
  definition, 23
  gestational, 24
  prevalence, 14
  treatment goals, 189
Diarrhea, 123
Diet soda, 128
Dietitians, 185
Dining out, 125
Dipeptidyl-peptidase-4
  inhibitors, 37
Dizziness, 124
Dolson, Laura, 120
Donaldson, Blake, 10
Dopamine receptor
  agonist, 34
DPP-4 inhibitors, 37
Drugs for diabetes, 29
  alpha-glucosidase
    inhibitors, 33
  bromocriptine, 34
  colesevelam, 36
  dipeptidyl-peptidase-4
    inhibitors, 37
  GLP-1 analogues, 39
  insulins, 42
  meglitinides, 45
  metformin, 46
  pramlintide, 48
  sulfonylureas, 50
  thiazolidinediones, 52

E

Eades, Mary Dan, 10

Eades, Michael R., 10
Eloff, Jennifer, 120
Endocrinologist, 186
Energy balance
  equation, 142
Evans, Frank, 10
Exenatide, 39
Exercise, 157
  aerobic activity, 166
  and diabetes, 171
  and heart health, 161
  and hypoglycemia, 173
  and insulin resistance, 162
  benefits, 158
  effect on weight loss, 160,
    161
  if markedly obese, 179
  metabolic effects, 159
  miscellaneous benefits,
    162
  recommendations, 163,
    164
  strength training, 165
  warnings for diabetics, 172
  weight management, 162
  with joint or back pain,
    183

F

Fat
  saturated, 11, 188
Fatigue, 122
**Fish, choose one to
  cook**, 125
FitDay, 130
Fitness, 161
Fitness, defined, 158
Free will, 145

G

Gastric inhibitory polypeptide, 37
Glimiperide, 50
Glinides, 45
Glipizide, 50
Glitazones, 52
GLP-1, 39
GLP-1 analogues, 39
Glucagon-like peptide-1, 37, 39
Glucose tablets, 58, 174
Glucose, blood
    averages in non-diabetic, 22
    Dr. Parker's treatment goals, 26
    test device inaccuracy, 28
    treatment goals, 25, 26
    venous versus capillary, 27
Glyburide, 50
Glyset, 33

H

Habits, starting new, 146
Harvey, William, 10
Hemoglobin A1c
    to diagnose diabetes & prediabetes, 24
    treatment goal, 26
Hirsch, James, 20
Holidays, 129, 137
Hunger management, 129
Hyperinsulinemia, 19
Hypoglycemia, 55, 58
    definition, 58
    drugs that cause, 61
    management options, 59
    symptoms, 58
    treatment, 58
    unawareness, 59
Hypoglycemia unawareness, 59

I

Induction flu, 122
Insulin
    formulations to treat diabetes, 42
    functions, 17, 20
Insulin resistance, 19, 162
Insulin secretagogues, 45

J

Januvia, 37

K

Ketogenic diet
    adverse effects, 70, 79, 121
Ketone bodies, 66
Ketones, 56
Keys, Ancel, 67, 144

L

Leg cramps, 122
Liraglutide, 39
Low blood sugar. *See* Hypoglycemia
Low Carb Friends, 120

M

Macronutrients in KMD, 73
Meals, typical for KMD, 93
Medical clearance, 170

Medications for diabetes.
  See Drugs for diabetes
Mediterranean diet
  definition, 68
  health benefits, 11, 67
Meglitinides, 45
Mercury in fish, 75
Metabolic syndrome, 64
Metformin, 46
Miglitol, 33
Motivation, 140

N

Nateglinide, 45
Neuropathy, 173, 176
NutritionData website,
  130

O

Obesity
  childhood, 15
Onglyza, 37
Overweight
  childhood, 15

P

Pancreas
  beta cell burn out, 19
  insulin secretion, 17
Parties, 137
Pedometers, 181
Pennington, Alfred, 10
Physical activity. *See*
  Exercise
Pioglitazone, 52
Pramlintide, 48
Prandin, 45
Precose, 33
Prediabetes

definition, 14, 23
prevalence, 14

R

Recipes, online sources,
  120
Recipes, special, 109
Record-keeping, 130
Repaglinide, 45
Retinopathy, 172
Rollo, John, 10, 63
Rosiglitazone, 52

S

Saxagliptin, 37
SELF-NutritionData, 130
Shopping, 124
Sitagliptin, 37
SparkPeople, 131
Spices
  Mediterranean, 78
Starlix, 45
Strength training, 165
Sulfonylureas, 50
Supplements
  recommended, 73
Sweet cravings, 128
Symlin, 48

T

Tanner, Thomas, 10
Target heart rate, 182
Taubes, Gary, 143, 144
Tea, 78
Thiazolidinediones, 52
Treatment goals, 186, 189

V

Vernon, Mary C., 10
Victoza, 39
Vildagliptin, 37
Vinaigrette, 94

W

Weight loss, 139

Weight loss goal, 148
Weight training, 165
WelChol, 36
Westman, Eric, 10
Willpower, 145

Y

Yogurt, 88

About the Author

Dr. Steve Parker is an Internal Medicine specialist with over two decades' experience treating people with diabetes and prediabetes. He's a leading medical expert on the Mediterranean diet and author of the award-winning *Advanced Mediterranean Diet: Lose Weight, Feel Better, Live Longer*. He lives with his wife and children in Arizona, U.S.A .

14718749R00115

Made in the USA
Charleston, SC
27 September 2012